NANOBIOTECHNOLOGY IN MOLECULAR DIAGNOSTICS

Current Techniques and Applications

By

Prof. K.K. Jain
MD, FRACS, FFPM
Jain PharmaBiotech
Basel, Switzerland

🌐 *horizon bioscience*

Copyright © 2006
Horizon Bioscience
32 Hewitts Lane
Wymondham
Norfolk NR18 0JA
U.K.

www.horizonbioscience.com

British Library Cataloguing-in-Publication Data

A catalogue record for this book is available from the British Library

ISBN: 1-904933-17-3

Printed and bound in Great Britain

AUTHOR'S BIOGRAPHY

Professor K. K. Jain is a neurologist/neurosurgeon by training and has been working in the biotechnology/biopharmaceuticals industry for several years. He received graduate training in both Europe and USA, has held academic positions in several countries and is a Fellow of the Faculty of Pharmaceutical Medicine of the Royal Colleges of UK. Currently he is a consultant at Jain PharmaBiotech. Prof. Jain is the author of over 350 publications including 11 books and 44 special reports, which have covered important areas in biotechnology, gene therapy and biopharmaceuticals. His publications include several articles on nanobiotechnology.

TABLE OF CONTENTS

TABLES

FIGURES

ABBREVIATIONS

Aβ	Amyloid beta
AFM	atomic force microscopy
ATP	adenosine triphosphate
bDNA	branched DNA
CGH	comparative genomic hybridization
ds	double stranded
DNA	deoxyribonucleic acid
ELISA	enzyme-linked immunosorbent assay
FISH	fluorescent in situ hybridization
FITC	fluorescein isothiocyanate
FRET	fluorescence energy transfer
GFP	green fluorescent protein
HCV	hepatitis C virus
HBV	hepatitis B virus
LC	liquid chromatography
MAbs	monoclonal antibodies
MRI	magnetic resonance imaging
MS	mass spectrometry
Nm	nanometer
PCR	polymerase chain reaction
QD	quantum dot
RLS	resonance light scattering
RNA	ribonucleic acid
rRNA	reporter RNA
RT	reverse transcriptase
ss	single stranded
SNP	single nucleotide polymorphism
SPR	surface plasmon resonance

PREFACE

Molecular diagnostics has been evolving rapidly during the past decade and has an impact on the practice of medicine as well as many other applications including drug discovery. Advances in biotechnology have been incorporated into molecular diagnostics. There has been a distinct trend in miniaturization with development of biochips and microfluidics. This trend has continued with the development of nanotechnology. Nanotechnologies are now being applied to molecular diagnostics to refine and extend the limits of detection. As the introductory chapter on molecular diagnostics shows, there are a large number of technologies and only a fraction of these have yet been affected by introduction of nanobiotechnology. There is a tremendous scope for further development.

This book gives an introduction of nanobiotechnology relevant to molecular diagnostics, a field that has been termed nanodiagnostics. Current state of development of nanodiagnostic technologies including nanobiochips and nanobiosensors is reviewed. Besides important applications in clinical diagnostics, the role of molecular diagnostics in drug discovery is also described.

This book was derived and expanded from the special report on nanobiotechnology by the author. The voluminous literature relevant to this topic was reviewed and 180 selected references are included in the bibliography. It will be useful for those developing nanobiotechnology, clinical laboratories, researchers in molecular diagnostics and scientists involved in drug discovery in the pharmaceutical industry. Financiers of nanotechnology have a scientific interest in the new developments and this book will be a source of useful information including development of technologies in the commercial sector.

K. K. Jain MD

Basel, Switzerland

November 2005

1. BASICS OF MOLECULAR DIAGNOSTICS

Abstract

Clinical application of molecular technologies to elucidate, diagnose and monitor human diseases is referred to as molecular diagnosis. Basics of molecular diagnostic technologies are described as an introduction to application of nanobiotechnologies for refining the tests. One example is molecular labels. Many types of nucleic acids require a secondary detection technology, e.g. a label, because a nucleic acid does not have intrinsic properties that are useful for direct high-sensitivity detection. Currently available labeling technologies have limited sensitivity and efficacy, which can be improved by nanoparticle technologies.

Introduction

Clinical application of molecular technologies to elucidate, diagnose and monitor human diseases is referred to as molecular diagnosis. It usually refers to the use of nucleic acid technologies that use DNA, RNA (ribonucleic acid), genes or proteins as bases for diagnostic tests. In a broader sense molecular diagnostics also includes the use of non-nucleic acid technologies such as monoclonal antibodies and enzyme-linked immunosorbent assay (ELISA). The historical evolution of molecular diagnostics relevant to nanobiotechnology is shown in Table 1-1.

Table 1-1: Historical evolution of molecular diagnostics

Year	Landmark/ Reference
1909	Phoebus Levene, an American chemist studying yeast, discovered deoxyribose – the D in DNA. In 1920, he identified the chemical bases of genome – adenine, cytosine, guanine and thymine
1920	The expression "Genom" used in German for the haploid chromosome set," which, together with the pertinent protoplasm, specifies the material foundations of the species
1944	DNA shown to carry genetic code in pneumococci (Avery 1944)
1953	Identification of the double-stranded structure of the DNA (Watson and Crick 1953)
1969	Discovery of in-situ hybridization for gene location by labeled RNA probes (Gall & Pardue 1969)

1975	Monoclonal antibody (MAb) technology (Köhler & Milstein 1975)
1980s	DNA probes: segments of DNA labeled with radioactive markers
1985	Discovery of polymerase chain reaction (Mullis et al 1986)
1986	Development of fluorescent in situ hybridization (FISH) technique (Pinkel et al 1986)
1988	DNA biosensor: electrochemical detection of DNA was carried out by the use of a fluoride ion selective electrode and stripping voltammetry (Downs et al 1988)
1990	First publication on in situ polymerase chain reaction (Haase et al 1990)
1991	Synthesis of DNA on a silicon chip – birth of the biochip (Fodor et al 1991).
1991	Wedding of molecular biology and cytogenetics and molecular cytogenetics (Lichter et al 1991)
1992	Branched DNA technology used to quantify HIV levels (Urdea et al 1993)
1992	Discovery of aptamers – single-stranded DNA molecules (Bock et al 1992)
1993	First publication on real-time PCR (Higuchi et al 1993)
1994	Potential of use of nanotechnology for biosensors (Sleytr et al 1994)
1995	Applications of proteomics (PROTEins expressed by a genOME) in molecular diagnostics
1998	Discovery of Locked Nucleic Acids (LNA), a novel class of DNA analogues, with potential applications in molecular diagnostics (Kumar et al 1998)
2005	X-ray crystallography used to determine the 3D structures of nearly all the possible sequences of DNA at atomic level and create a map of DNA structure, facilitating the study of gene function.

© Jain PharmaBiotech

There are over six hundred such diagnostic systems. Detailed description of molecular diagnostic technologies is given elsewhere (Jain 2005). Many new technologies such as nanotechnology have been used to refine molecular diagnostics. The focus of this report is on application of nanobiotechnology to molecular diagnosis and basic techniques of molecular diagnostics will be described in this chapter. Polymerase chain reaction (PCR) is the most important of these technologies. There are several modifications of PCR and non-PCR diagnostic technologies as well.

The polymerase chain reaction

The polymerase chain reaction (PCR) is a method of nucleic acid analysis for producing large amounts of a specific DNA fragment of a defined sequence and length from a small amount of a complex template. It can selectively amplify a single molecule of DNA or RNA several million-fold in a few hours. Use of this technology enables the detection and analysis of specific gene sequences in a patient's sample without cloning. Analyses can be performed on even a few cells from body fluids or in a drop of blood. Thus, PCR eliminates the need to prepare large amounts of DNA from tissue samples. PCR has revolutionized molecular diagnostics. Apart from laboratory diagnosis, it has affected genomics and biotechnology as well.

Basic principles of PCR

PCR is based on the enzymatic amplification of a fragment of DNA that is flanked by two "primers"--short oligonucleotides that hybridize to the opposite strands of the target sequence and then prime synthesis of the complementary DNA sequence by DNA polymerase (an enzyme). The chain reaction is a three-step process – denaturation, annealing, and extension – that is repeated in several cycles. At each stage of the process, the number of copies is doubled from two to four, to eight, and so on. The reactions are controlled by changing the temperature using a special heat-stable Taq polymerase. After 20 cycles, roughly 1 million copies exist, or enough material to detect the desired DNA by conventional means such as color reaction.

RNA can also be studied by making a DNA copy of the RNA using the enzyme reverse transcriptase. Such an approach enables the study of mRNA in cells that use the molecule to synthesize specific proteins or the detection of the genome of RNA viruses. PCR has been fully automated via use of thermal cycling. It is a fast, sensitive, and specific test with applications in diagnosis of various diseases described in following chapters.

Target selection

Several strategies are available for selecting a genetic target to be amplified so as to detect an infectious disease organism. For example, genes that contain both conserved and variable sequence regions may be targeted. In such a case, specificity may be obtained either at the amplification (primer) or detection (probe) stage. The target may also consist of a virulent gene that is uniquely responsible for distinguishing pathogenic from closely related nonpathogenic strains, types, or species.

Detection of amplified DNA

The first detection methods used with PCR were radioactively labeled probes that identified specific amplified sequences. With improvements in specificity, it became possible to visualize amplified DNA of the predicted size directly by examining its fluorescence after staining. Probes have now been converted to nonisotopic colorimetric systems. In another approach, the probe is a "reverse" component (bound to a membrane) and "captures" a specific allele or a sequence variant if it is present in the amplified DNA.

An alternative to probe-based detection system relies on labeled primers and strives for perfect target specificity in the amplification reaction. This process is straightforward if the target gene differs from the unintended targets by a deletion or gene rearrangement. Using the Duchenne muscular dystrophy gene deletions as a model, researchers have now automated this method. It should prove highly useful in forensic investigations for rapid analysis of amplified targets that differ in length, such as variable number tandem repeat (VNTR) loci.

In general, nonradioactive detection systems fall into two classes – direct and indirect – based on the detectability of the label. In most indirect detection methods, the primary label (e.g., biotin) is identified through its interaction with a secondary system that contains a detectable reporter group. Various techniques for direct detection of nucleic acids include the following:

- Direct enzymatic detection, which requires the construction of enzyme DNA conjugates.

- Fluorescent detection, which depends on the ability to synthesize fluorescent DNA. This technique may emerge as the detection technology of choice in future PCR systems.

- Chemiluminescent detection via direct attachment of chemiluminescent labels (e.g., acridium esters and isoluminol derivatives) to synthetic nucleotides.

DNA sequencing and molecular diagnostics

DNA sequencing was initially used only for research purposes but has now become a routine tool in molecular diagnostics. Several research and clinical laboratories are now using DNA/RNA sequencing technology in the following molecular diagnostic applications:

- HIV resistance sequence analysis

- HCV genotyping

- Microbial identification

- Genetic diseases

- Molecular epidemiological studies: genotyping of microorganisms and predisposition testing in cancer.

Novel PCR methods

Hundreds of modifications of the basic PCR have been developed to enhance the method beyond the original design. PCR-based techniques are used to quantify nucleic acids, amplify RNAs, characterize genomes and perform DNA fingerprinting. An important example is real-time PCR.

Real-time PCR systems

Some of the limitations of end-point PCR have been addressed in real-time PCR systems, a number of which are now on the market. These systems offer many general technical advantages, including reduced probabilities of variability and contamination, as well as online monitoring and the lack of need for post reaction analyses. Further, some of these systems were developed with contemporary applications such as quantitative PCR, multiplexing, and high-throughput (HT) analysis in mind. In addition, application of real-time PCR has provided significant methodological benefits and improved patient outcomes. In the decade following the first publication on real-time PCR, thousands of papers have appeared in the literature. The range of application is immense and has been partially fulfilled by the availability of lower-cost instruments and reagents. Real-time quantitative PCR is a highly sensitive method that is especially useful for evaluating RNA fingerprints obtained from short interfering RNA (siRNA) experiments and for scientists using RNA interference (RNAi) for mapping cellular pathways.

There are currently five main chemistries used for the detection of PCR product during real-time PCR: DNA binding fluorophores, 5' endonuclease, adjacent linear and hairpin oligoprobes, and the self-fluorescing amplicons. In real-time quantitative PCR techniques, signals (generally fluorescent) are monitored as they are generated and are tracked after they rise above background but before the reaction reaches a plateau. Initial template levels can be calculated by analyzing the shape of the curve or by determining when the signal rises above some threshold value.

Of the important applications is the combination of real-time PCR with either laser capture microdissection or nucleic acids from paraffin-fixed archival samples or whole-transcript amplification from very small numbers of cells. It will be possible to measure gene expression or DNA copy number in specific cell types that are available only in a small quantity. Real-time Q-PCR can be applied to analysis of clinical samples to help stratification of patients in personalized medicine approach. The safety of cell-derived biological compounds or quantification of retrovirus-like particles will be enhanced with real-time Q-PCR. It will also be useful for identification of potential contaminants during the production of recombinant monoclonal antibodies (MAbs) for therapeutic use. Combining techniques for sorting fetal cells or DNA from the maternal circulation with Q-PCR will enable early minimally invasive prenatal diagnosis of numerous congenital disorders. Confirmation of expression levels of selected genes from microarray experiments will continue to be conducted using real-time PCR methods. Real-time PCR can be incorporated in the development of highly specific assays that can be performed in the field for use in screening for evidence of biological weapons.

Non-PCR nucleic acid amplification methods

A number of non-PCR technologies for nucleic acid amplifications have emerged that offer advantages for particular applications. The advantages include added convenience and cost-effectiveness as no thermal cycler is needed. They often require minimal sample preparation as they rely on a series of steps to add reagents. Many of these are complementary rather than competitive to PCR. Some of these technologies are described in the following text.

Linked Linear Amplification

Linked Linear Amplification (LLA) is a new nucleic acid amplification method that uses multiple cycles of primer extension reactions. The presence of nonreplicable elements in LLA primers renders primer extension products unusable as templates for further amplification, leading to linear accumulation of products. Through the use of nested primers, linear reactions can be "linked", providing total amplification yields comparable to those obtained by PCR. The LLA model predicts (a) that amplification yield will approach that of PCR as the number of primers increases and (b) that the unique composition of LLA products will give lower carryover amplification efficiency compared with PCR. LLA is a robust target amplification method with an advantage over PCR that it is more resistant to false results caused by carryover amplicon contamination.

Transcription mediated amplification

Transcription mediated amplification (TMA) is an isothermal nucleic-acid-based method that can amplify RNA or DNA targets a billion-fold in less than one hour's time. This system is useful for detecting the presence of *M. tuberculosis* and *C. trachomatis*.

Developed at Gen-Probe, TMA technology uses two primers and two enzymes: RNA polymerase and reverse transcriptase. One primer contains a promoter sequence for RNA polymerase. In the first step of amplification, this primer hybridizes to the target rRNA at a defined site. Reverse transcriptase creates a DNA copy of the target rRNA by extension from the 3'end of the promoter primer. The RNA in the resulting RNA:DNA duplex is degraded by the RNase activity of the reverse transcriptase. Next, a second primer binds to the DNA copy. A new strand of DNA is synthesized from the end of this primer by reverse transcriptase, creating a double-stranded DNA molecule. RNA polymerase recognizes the promoter sequence in the DNA template and initiates transcription. Each of the newly synthesized RNA amplicons reenters the TMA process and serves as a template for a new round of replication. The amplicons produced in these reactions are detected by a specific gene probe in hybridization protection assay, a chemiluminescence detection format.

Rapid analysis of gene expression

Current techniques for analysis of gene expression either monitor one gene at a time, for example northern hybridization or RT-PCR methods, or are designed for the simultaneous analysis of thousands of genes, for example microarray hybridization or serial analysis of gene expression. To provide a flexible, intermediate scale alternative, a PCR-based method RAGE (rapid analysis of gene expression) has been developed which allows expression changes to be determined in either a directed search of known genes, or an undirected survey of unknown genes. A single set of reagents and reaction conditions allows analyses of most genes in any eukaryote. The method is useful for assaying on the order of tens to hundreds of genes in multiple samples. Control experiments indicate reliable detection of changes in gene expression 2-fold and greater, and sensitivity of detection better than 1 in 10,000. This technology has been applied to investigate the changes in gene expression in human cells following treatment with a carcinogen and to determine the changes in large numbers of genes in early stage breast cancer. These molecular "signatures" of cancer may then be used to determine which tumors are likely to be responsive to chemotherapy.

WAVE nucleic acid fragment analysis system

Transgenomics' proprietary WAVE Nucleic Acid Fragment Analysis System has been designed and optimized to use the DNASep cartridge for separating (ds or ss) DNA. WAVE is also commonly known as DHPLC (denaturing high performance liquid chromatography). The system can easily resolve PCR products that have small differences in their lengths. The WAVE System is based on the company's proprietary micro-bead technology. The patented micro-beads are packed into proprietary DNASep separation column, which is the key component of WAVE System. Each microbead has specific surface chemistry that interacts with DNA molecules. The DNA molecules are then selectively separated from the micro-beads with a mixture of liquid reagents. The system is computer controlled and contains the proprietary software WAVEMAKER, which predicts analytical parameters with a high accuracy for optimal fragment separation and mutational analysis. The WAVE HS System incorporates fluorescence detection to expand the high-sensitivity in analysis of nucleic acid fragments. Advantages of WAVE include high sensitive, accuracy (can detect as little as 1 copy of a mutated allele in 100 wild type copies), speed, cost-effectiveness and versatility (enables many fluorescent labels to be utilized). Because of this versatility, the WAVE System can essentially replace the use of traditional gel electrophoresis in the molecular biology laboratory. Applications include the following:

- Mutation screening

- Polymorphic marker mapping

- Linkage analysis

- Cancer epidemiology

- Population studies

- Forensic and paternity analysis (STR)

- Loss of heterozygosity (LOH)

WAVE analyzes previously identified genes for any variations, changes or mutations. Mutations discovered by DHPLC may provide researchers with critical information about the cause, onset and progression of certain diseases. Scanning for mutations in genes with the WAVE System relies on the specific binding of complementary strands of the DNA double helix. If a mutation exists, a DNA heteroduplex (pairing of different strands) is formed and the binding is less "tight." High temperatures can be used to denature (melt) the DNA double helix. If a mutation exists, the melting temperature of the heteroduplex will be lower. Partially melted DNA can be easily separated from unmelted DNA homoduplexes (pairings of similar strands) containing no mutation. WAVE technology is ideal for the design of new tests for inherited diseases, particularly those characterized by a variety of potential mutation sites dispersed across large or complex genes. Since the WAVE System detects any mutation within a particular DNA fragment, there is no need to design and optimize a specific probe- or primer-based assay for each individual mutation.

Rolling circle amplification technology

Rolling circle amplification technology (RCAT), a proprietary amplification process developed by Molecular Staging Inc, has significant advantages in terms of sensitivity, multiplexing, dynamic range and scalability. The steps of this procedure are:

1. A short DNA probe anneals to a target DNA of interest, such as the DNA of a pathogenic organism or a human gene containing a deleterious mutation. The probe then acts as a primer for a Rolling Circle Amplification reaction (see 2).

2. The free end of the probe anneals to a small circular DNA template. A DNA polymerase (white oval) is added to extend the primer.

3. The DNA polymerase extends the primer continuously around the circular DNA template generating a long DNA product that consists of many repeated copies of the circle.

4. By the end of the reaction, the polymerase generates many thousands of copies of the circular template, with the chain of copies tethered to the original target DNA. This allows for spatial resolution of target and rapid amplification of the signal. The use of forward and reverse primers can change the above linear amplification reaction into an exponential mode.

RCAT can achieve the following:

- Detect single target molecules or "analytes".

- Amplify signals from proteins as well as DNA and RNA.

- Pinpoint the location of molecules that have been amplified on a solid surface (in situ analysis/ biochips) since, unlike PCR, the amplified product remains attached to the target molecule.

- Measure many different targets simultaneously.

- Improve the ease and accuracy of quantification.

- Simplify haplotype identification through phasing.

- Increase sensitivity with up to 10^{12} -fold amplification in one hour.

- Amplify DNA templates that vary in length from 1 base pair to over 100 kilobases.

- Obviate the need for the time-consuming and expensive steps of thermal cycling currently.

- Analyze targets in solution or solid phase.

Technologies for signal amplification

Signal amplification implies direct detection of nucleic acids without target amplification. Various technologies for signal amplification are shown in Table 1-2.

Table 1-2: Technologies for signal amplification

Technology/company	Principle/ method	Applications
Q beta replicase system/ Vysis	Amplification of the signal of the probe is quantitatively because of linear amplification.	Quantification of HIV-1 mRNA as targets, with limit of about 104 mRNA molecules.
3DNA dendrimer signal amplification/Genisphere Inc	The arborescent structure of dendritic molecules allows them to be readily labeled with numerous fluorescent compounds.	Enables detection of extremely low concentrations of analytes in diagnostic assays.
Hybridization signal amplification method/ Hamilton Thorne Bioscience	A self-assembling, structurally defined nanostructure, comprised of short ligand-derived nucleic acids and multivalent anti-ligand molecules, is introduced to bind to the target-bound probes.	Alternative to enzymatic amplification systems in situations where simplicity and speed are primary criteria in assay design.
Signal mediated amplification of RNA technology (SMART)/ Cytocell	Two oligonucleotide probes hybridize to a specific target sequence and then to each other forming a three-way junction	Ideal for pharmacogenomic applications where large numbers of patients are required to be genotyped
Invader operating system /Third Wave Technologies	Based on a "perfect match" enzyme-substrate reaction.	Several applications in molecular diagnostics.

Hybrid Capture (HC) technology/Digene Corporation	It uses antibody capture and chemiluminescence for signal detection.	HC technology achieves clinically relevant levels of detection.
Branched DNA (bDNA)/ Bayer	Amplifies signals in a controlled manner so that the number of target molecules is not increased.	Quantitative assays to detect HBV DNA, HCV RNA, and HIV-1 RNA in the plasma.
Tyramide signal amplification (TMA)/ PerkinElmer	Amplifies signals with catalyzed reporter-deposition technique.	ELISA, immunohistochemistry, in situ hybridization, etc.

© Jain PharmaBiotech

3 DNA dendrimer signal amplification

The name "dendrimer", derived from the Greek word for "tree", suggests the unusual structure of this highly branched molecule. As a class, dendrimers are complex, branched molecules built from interconnected natural or synthetic monomeric subunits. A 3DNA dendrimer is constructed from DNA monomers – as the name "3DNA" indicates. Each 3DNA monomer is composed of two DNA strands that share a region of sequence complementarity located in the central portion of each strand. When the two strands anneal to form the monomer the resulting structure has a central double-stranded "waist" bordered by four single-stranded "arms". This "waist" plus "arms" structure comprises the basic 3DNA monomer.

The arborescent structure of dendritic molecules makes them extremely useful for the development of nucleic acid diagnostics as signal amplification tools. Further, due to the relatively large size of nucleic acid molecules, nucleic acid dendrimers could be readily labeled with numerous fluorescent compounds and/or protein moieties. DNA dendrimers provide a generic method for amplifying signal and have general utility in nucleic acid blot assays. Dendritic DNA molecules (3DNA) could be readily labeled with numerous fluorescent compounds. Specificity to various DNA sequences is conferred to the dendrimers by hybridizing and covalently crosslinking oligonucleotides to the single-stranded surface of the dendrimers. Genisphere Inc is currently investigating applications of the dendrimer in Southern, Northern, and Western blots, fluorescent in-situ hybridization (FISH), and flow fluorescence assays. In a hybridization reaction, signal intensity is determined by the amount of label that can be localized at the reaction site. The 3DNA dendrimers in all of Genisphere kits are labeled with an average of at least 200 labels (more in some kits). The dendrimer carries this number of labels with it every time it hybridizes to a complementary molecule. The result is up to a 200-fold passive enhancement of signal intensity.

A versatile and strong signal amplification method is based on activities of a DNA polymerase to generate high concentrations of pyrophosphate (PPi), which is catalyzed by nucleotide extension and excision activities of a DNA polymerase on an oligonucleotide cassette. The signal is generated upon enzymatic conversion of PPi to ATP and ATP levels subsequently detected with firefly luciferase. Bioluminescence produced by an oligonucleotide cassette consisting of just two polymerase reaction sites is sufficient to detect them at low attomole levels. The attachment of a large number of these oligonucleotide cassettes to DNA dendrimers enables the detection of such polyvalent substrate molecules at low zeptomole concentrations. The extent of signal amplification obtained with dendrimer substrates is comparable to exponential target amplifications provided by nucleic acid amplification methods. The attachment of such PPi-generating dendritic DNA platforms to ligands that mediate target recognition would potentially permit detection of extremely low concentrations of analytes in diagnostic assays.

Hybridization signal amplification method

Hybridization signal amplification method (HSAM), developed by Hamilton Thorne Bioscience, is an elegantly simple signal amplification method that takes advantage of some of the unique structural capabilities of nucleic acids. It is a companion to ramification amplification method (RAM). Conceptually, HSAM can be thought of as a variation on traditional probe network signal amplification schemes, updated by incorporation of cutting-edge nanostructure concepts. HSAM can be used to detect nucleic acids, proteins, or other small molecules that might typically be measured by immunoassay.

In practice, a ligand-derived probe (nucleic acid or antibody) reacts specifically with the target molecule. Then, a self-assembling, structurally defined nanostructure, comprised of short ligand-derived nucleic acids and multivalent anti-ligand molecules, is introduced to bind to the target-bound probes.

Components of the nanostructure can be derived from a variety of signal-generating moieties – e.g., fluorescent tags for direct detection or enzymes that can themselves generate detectable moieties in an indirect fashion – to suit specific applications. The nanostructure provides a many-fold greater surface area for supporting detection moieties than the probe molecule itself.

HSAM is an attractive alternative to enzymatic amplification systems in situations where simplicity and speed are primary criteria in assay design. It should be particularly useful in solid phase or microarray types of applications where enzymatic amplification/detection can be cumbersome. HSAM also expands the signal amplification capabilities beyond nucleic acids to include proteins and other small antigens in the same analytical system. RAM and HSAM (Hybridization Signal Amplification Method), represent the next generation of technology after PCR. RAM and HSAM have significant advantages in sensitivity, multiplexing, quantification, and dynamic range over older amplification methods and offer real-time, super-exponential amplification. These technologies are capable of detecting, quantifying and analyzing all classes of biomolecules, including DNA, RNA and proteins. The high sensitivity is singularly appropriate for detection down to the levels of single cells and even single molecules (rare events). This method is also used with extreme simplicity and sensitivity to detect viruses and bacteria in clinical specimens. In-situ (on a slide) detection of multiple viral sequences in cells is also possible using RAM technology. Most importantly, much of the work performed with RAM and HSAM has been done on actual clinical samples and not in idealized research laboratory conditions. Other advantages of RAM and HSAM over current amplification techniques include:

- The platform offers high specificity and reproducibility.

- Multiplexing: Simultaneous measurement is possible of many protein analytes or DNA sequences. The objective is rapid and low cost analysis.

- This technology can quantify target analytes or sequences over a wide dynamic range and with an accuracy that is considerably above current methods.

- Simple preparation and high throughput: Some of the formats require only one step to perform the assay, bringing DNA analysis on level with the ease and low cost of common clinical tests.

- The RAM/HSAM platform is highly effective in solution, on solid surfaces such as biochips, in microfluidics, with a wide range of solid supports and as a slide based cell assay.

Signal mediated amplification of RNA technology

Signal mediated amplification of RNA technology (SMART) has been developed by Cytocell. The assay consists of two oligonucleotide probes that hybridize to a specific target sequence and, only then, to each other forming a three-way junction. One probe (template for the RNA signal) contains a non-functional single-stranded T7 RNA polymerase promoter sequence. This promoter sequence is made double-stranded (hence functional) by DNA polymerase, allowing T7 RNA polymerase to generate a target-dependent RNA signal which is measured by an enzyme-linked oligosorbent assay. This method also enables the generation of signals from *E. coli* samples without prior extraction of nucleic acid, showing that for some targets, sample purification may not be required. The assay will be quantitative for infectious disease agents: the level of signal relates directly to the amount of target and therefore to the number of organisms in the original sample. Currently the assay requires no thermal cycling, and can be carried out in a single well. Finally, the assay will be relatively easy to automate, making it suitable for high throughput screening for detection of multiple genetic variants with known sequences. This makes it ideal for pharmacogenomic applications where large numbers of patients are required to be genotyped in clinical trials or in a clinical laboratory where an automatable assay is disease detection is needed.

Direct molecular analysis without amplification

The Trilogy™ Platform (US Genomics) is founded on the belief that direct analysis of single biological molecules is the key to the next generation of revolutionary technologies. US Genomics is developing technologies that can directly analyze individual molecules of DNA, RNA and proteins, without PCR amplification. The process of direct analysis by the Trilogy platform begins with the isolation of target material (DNA, RNA or protein) from a biological source, followed by fluorescently tagging the sample material at specific sites of interest (e.g. a nucleotide sequence motif or protein epitope). The sample is then injected into the microfluidic system of the Trilogy Instrument, and the sample passes through an interrogation region consisting of several laser spots. Each molecule is detected by the laser excitation of the fluorescent tags on the molecule. Thousands of molecules pass through the system per minute.

Trilogy Analysis replaces traditional molecular biology techniques, hampered by the need for amplification and bulk fluorescence, with the accuracy and sensitivity of direct measurements based on single molecules. Direct analysis on the Trilogy platform utilizes color coincidence counting to detect and quantify individual biomolecules that have been fluorescently labeled, then directed by proprietary microfluidics to the Trilogy's multi-color laser interrogation and detection region. Individual molecules are monitored by color fluorescence, and color coincidence is used to distinguish and quantify true molecular events, lending the system high specificity and strong signal-to-noise. Additional advantages of the platform include:

- Sensitivity in the femtomolar range.

- No need for amplification (e.g. PCR) or enzymatic procedures, eliminating a major source of cost and bias.

- Small sample material requirements.

- Flexibility across sample types (e.g. DNA, RNA and protein) and assays.

Trilogy Analysis is compatible with a wide range of sample types and assays. Quantification of molecules of interest such as RNA transcripts is accomplished by direct dual-labeling of RNA with fluorescently labeled oligonucleotides, eliminating the need for reverse transcription or PCR. Detection of specific nucleotide sequences such as SNP polymorphisms is achieved through probe hybridization or an extension reaction. And interactions between two fluorescently labeled molecules (e.g. protein-protein, protein-DNA, protein-small molecule) can easily be detected and quantified at the molecular level, making biochemical characterization of such interactions a rapid, accurate and convenient process.

In DirectLinear™ Analysis, DNA molecules up to megabases in length are tagged with specific fluorophores and pass through a proprietary microfluidics system which stretches them to their full length, causing them to pass through and be read by the laser excitation and detection region in a linear fashion. The data generated is equivalent to a genetic "barcode" representing the spatial map of the fluorescent tags along the DNA. Each genomic barcode is unique to a specific individual or organism.

DirectLinear™ Analysis has numerous potential applications in life science research and drug discovery and development. Entire genomes of novel organisms can be mapped nearly instantaneously, inviting comparison with known genomes and allowing researchers to focus on conserved regions or novel genomic features. Genetic differences between two samples or populations can readily be detected by comparing differences in barcode patterns, allowing the rapid identification of polymorphisms associated with disease or adverse drug response. Rapid genomic mapping of microbial organisms will have great utility in research and diagnostics in infectious disease, as well as in biodefense. Finally, rapid, low-cost access to each person's genomic information is the key to enabling molecular diagnostics and, ultimately, personalized medicine.

Molecular labels

Many types of nucleic acids require a secondary detection technology, e.g. a label, because a nucleic acid does not have intrinsic properties that are useful for direct high-sensitivity detection. Reasons for ultrasensitive nucleic acid detection include analysis of genetic material from single cells and single copy gene detection. Molecular labels provide the means for detecting and evaluating most biological interactions, such as those involving DNA, proteins, whole cells and pathogens. Currently available technologies have limited sensitivity and efficacy. Desirable characteristics of a label are stability, sensitivity of detection, speed and convenience of detection and low cost. No ideal label fulfilling all of these properties is available as yet. Better labels or detection reactions may enable an assay that requires fewer amplification cycles and eliminates the need for PCR. A selection of molecular labels and technologies for their detection is shown in Table 1-3. Nanoparticle technologies for molecular labeling will be described in later chapters. To make DNA technology attainable for routine diagnostics, several non-radioactive alternatives have been developed.

Table 1-3: Selected labels for nucleic acid detection

DNA labeling with digoxigenin
Non-isotopic labeling of DNA
Enzyme labels, e.g., acetate kinase
Microparticles, e.g., quantum dots
Nanoparticle technology
Microtransponder-based DNA diagnostics
Laboratory Multiple Analyte Profile
Multiple labels
Avidin or streptavidin reagents
Labeled dendrimers
DNA-tagged liposomes
Conjugate binding to label

Detection technologies for molecular labels

A vast array of different labels and assay strategies has been developed to meet the requirements of sensitivity, accuracy and convenience. Instruments for detection include: fluorescence and confocal microscopy, flow cytometry, laser scanning cytometry, fluorescence microplate analysis and biochips. The development of increasingly sensitive labels and detection equipment has seen a drastic improvement in the sensitivity of immunoassay systems, allowing an ever-increasing range of analytes to be measured accurately. Availability of fluorescence and labeling technologies has also a considerable impact on the development of nucleic acid-based diagnostics.

Fluorescence and chemiluminescence

In earlier years scientists tagged samples – whether nucleic acid, protein, cell, or tissue – with radioactive labels, and captured images on film. Safety concerns, convenience, and sensitivity, spurred the development of alternative techniques, and today, researchers can choose from a range of options, including fluorescence and chemiluminescence, in addition to autoradiography. Fluorescence occurs when light is absorbed from an external (excitation) source by a fluorescent molecule (fluorophore) and subsequently emitted. The cycle of excitation and emission will continue until the excitation source is turned off or the fluorophore is consumed in a chemical reaction. A fluorescent probe is any small molecule that that undergoes changes in one or more of its fluorescent properties as a result of noncovalent interaction with a protein or other macromolecular structure. There are many different fluorescent molecules, both naturally occurring and synthetic, each molecule having distinctive spectroscopic properties. This variety of molecules can be exploited to enable highly localized, sensitive detection of chemical reactions, for tagging and identification of molecular structures, for monitoring of cellular states, and even for monitoring multiple properties simultaneously. Due to their higher sensitivity than chromogenic dyes, the fluorescent probes can be used to effectively signal the presence of minute amounts of a specific protein, DNA or RNA without the hazards associated with radioactive labels.

Chemiluminescence is the production of visible light (luminescence) occurring as a result of a chemical reaction. It can be exploited as a labeling method in nucleic acid hybridization. Chemiluminescence is typically about 2 orders of magnitude more sensitive than fluorescence and more than 4 orders of magnitude more sensitive than chromogenic reactions.

Bioluminescence is light emitted by biological sources and has been used for diagnostics. Bacterial (lux) and eukaryotic (luc) luciferase genes are valuable as "reporters" of many endpoints of clinical concern. The development of new technologies for monitoring biological and chemical contaminants includes the use of genes encoding enzymes for bioluminescence as reporter systems. Applications of

17

the recombinant luciferase reporter phage concept now provide a sensitive approach for bacterial detection, viability, and sensitivity to antimicrobial agents. Moreover, a number of fusions of the lux and luc genes to stress inducible genes in different bacteria can allow a real-time measurement of gene expression and determination of cellular viability, and also constitute a new tool to detect toxic chemicals and their bioavailability.

Many of the technologies, which use fluorescence for label detection, are in development for both in vitro and in vivo diagnostics. They can offer equivalent, if not higher, sensitivity than isotope detection systems and have the added advantage of greater versatility, stability, and safe handling. Further, genetically encoded probes offer the possibility of biosensors for intracellular biochemistry, specifically localized targets, and protein-protein interactions. DNA-based fluorescent microarrays are becoming an increasingly important tool for studying gene expression, identifying new drug targets, and developing gene-based diagnostic protocols. Fluorescence detection systems include readers, probes, dyes, and reagents.

Molecular beacons

Molecular beacons were developed as an extension of the concept of fluorescently labeled oligonucleotides. The molecular beacon is a folded probe that gives no fluorescent signal in the folded position due to quenching of the label. Upon hybridization of the molecular beacon to the target sequence (amplicon RNA), the probe unfolds and the fluorescent label emits light. When the molecular beacon is away from its target sequence, the stem structure holds the fluorophore and the quenching groups together but the stem structure is pulled apart upon interaction with target DNA. During the PCR, molecular beacons bind to the synthesized DNA and the resulting level of fluorescence can be directly correlated with the target DNA. This is an improvement on measuring the amount of PCR products by treating the sample with intercalating fluorescent dyes which lack specificity. One of the first techniques to use molecular beacons was realtime PCR. Several innovations have been made in molecular beacons. Molecular beacons may be coupled to NASBA (nucleic acid sequence-based amplification).

Molecular beacons are able to discriminate alleles in real-time PCR assays of genomic DNA. This approach can be used to analyze any DNA sequence of moderate length with single base pair accuracy. Molecular beacons present a solution for the high-throughput screening of SNPs in homogenous assays using the PCR. The ability of molecular beacons to discriminate between sequences makes them an ideal tool for genetic screening and diagnostics. Molecular beacons are also moving into the biochip world.

Single-base mismatches can be detected using DNA microarrays in a format that does not require labeling of the sample (target) DNA. The method is based on disrupting fluorescence energy transfer (FRET) between a fluorophore attached to an immobilized DNA strand (probe) and a quencher-containing sequence that is complementary. Using this method with an oligonucleotide model system, single-base mismatches can successfully discriminate at levels greater than that observed using surface-immobilized molecular beacons. A pair of molecular beacons, one with a donor and the other with an acceptor fluorophore that hybridize to adjacent regions on the same mRNA target, result in FRET. Such a dual FRET molecular beacons approach provides a novel technique for sensitive RNA detection and quantification in living cells (Santangelo et al 2004).

The Green fluorescent protein

Certain marine organisms produce calcium-activated photoproteins that enable them to emit light for a variety of purposes, such as defense, feeding, breeding, etc. Even though there are many bioluminescent organisms in nature, only a few photoproteins have been isolated and characterized. The mechanism of emission of light is an internal chemical reaction. Because there is no need for excitation through external irradiation for the emission of bioluminescence, the signal produced has virtually no background, allowing for the detection of the proteins at extremely low levels. Thus photoproteins, aequorin, obelin, and the green fluorescent protein (GFP), are attractive labels for analytical applications. Of these GFP is the one most frequently used for bioanalysis.

GFP, obtained from the jellyfish Aequorea victoria has an amazing ability to generate a highly visible, efficiently emitting internal fluorophore. High-resolution crystal structures of GFP offer unprecedented opportunities to understand and manipulate the relation between protein structure and spectroscopic function. GFP has become well established as a marker of gene expression and protein targeting in intact cells and organisms. Mutagenesis and engineering of GFP into chimeric proteins are opening new vistas in physiological indicators, biosensors, and photochemical labels.

Enzyme labels and detection by fluorescence

The basis of most nucleic acid assays is exploitation of the specificity of base recognition (e.g., adenine for thymine) and the high binding constant of resulting duplexes. Competitive and noncompetitive amperometric immunoassays have been developed with enzymes as labels. The sensitivity of assays can be improved by using an enzyme label such as acetate kinase, which can be detected with higher sensitivity. Such an enzyme label can be detected down to a zeptomole level using a bioluminescent assay. ATP formed by the action of the enzyme label on the acetylphosphatase substrate is measured using a firefly luciferase reaction. The expressed enzyme and the gene for the bioluminescent luciferase class of enzymes are promising labels for nucleic acid detection. The gene can be manipulated to produce mutants that catalyze light at different wavelengths. The gene for the enzyme luciferase itself may be used rather than the product of the gene. This enables many enzyme molecules to be transcribed from an individual gene label, thus introducing a high amplification factor into the assay.

Fluorescent in situ hybridization

In situ hybridization has emerged as a powerful and versatile tool for the detection and localization of nucleic acid sequences within an intact cell, chromosome, or tissue preparation by means of labeled complementary sequences (in situ means in intact cells as opposed to gels or membranes). Development of in situ hybridization provided greater resolution than was possible via chromosomal banding. This technique may be used for the following purposes (Jain 2004):

- Identification of sites of gene expression.

- Analysis of the tissue distribution of transcription.

- Tracking of changes in specific mRNA synthesis.

- Chromosome labeling and mapping.

- Investigations of genetic alterations within the context of cell morphology and tissue architecture that hold particular importance in tumor pathology.

- Identification and localization of viral infection.

- Synthesis of histopathologic and molecular biologic data that are enormously important in diagnostic pathology.

The essential steps of the in situ hybridization procedure include preparation of the specimen, probe labeling, hybridization, and detection. Several methods are used for detection. Radiolabeled DNA probes, for example, have been used to define the chromosomal localization of a single copy of DNA sequences in metaphase chromosomes.

Fluorescent nucleotide labels are employed in fluorescent in situ hybridization (FISH) techniques, including the highly effective non-isotopic fluorescent hybridization approach. FISH has four components--target, probes, fluorescent detection, and visualization. A number of DNA probes, each labeled with a different fluorochrome, can be used in the same procedure so that separate loci can be identified and compared. Probes are hybridized to target DNA and tagged with a fluorochrome, either before or after hybridization. Numerous sources of these probes have been found, including oligonucleotides, PCR products, cDNA, genomic fragments contained in plasmids, bacteriophages, cosmids, and yeast artificial chromosomes (YACs).

The following principles underlie the FISH technology:

- If native DNA is denatured to a single-stranded configuration, incubation with specifically labeled DNA will result in complementary strand binding (hybridization) to form a double strand and to produce a localized appearance of a label at the chromosomal or intranuclear site where that DNA normally resides.

- In the same way, RNA will hybridize with a complementary or "antisense" strand of either RNA or DNA.

- Greater similarity between the strands leads to tighter bonding.

- Specific segments of DNA (genes or chromosomal regions) can be tagged directly with biotin or digoxigenin and then linked with a fluorescent label.

The advent of recombinant DNA technology has made it theoretically possible to detect a unique sequence anywhere in the genome. If the quantity of available DNA is limited, PCR amplification can be used to enhance the sample. In practice, probes typically consist of double-stranded cDNA cloned in plasmid vectors. If a fluorescent cDNA probe is denatured and then mixed with a large amount of denatured repetitive DNA, only the labeled nonrepetitive sequences in the probe anneal to the targets. FISH can locate more than one sequence at a time by using different colors of the "paint."

FISH has provided an additional tool by which to examine meiosis and events in the development of chromosomal abnormalities. It can be used to stain chromosomes in interphase nuclei, a process termed "interphase genetics", so as to study abnormalities in the chromosomes of nonproliferating cells and cells taken directly from tissue biopsies. This method requires a DNA probe that usually consists of a cloned portion of a genomic DNA containing both specific gene sequences and repetitive DNA. The probe is labeled with a fluorescent tag, and then the two strands of DNA are denatured. The labeled probe is mixed with an excess of unlabeled repetitive DNA sequences that bind to repetitive sequences in the probe, leaving only the specific sequences available for binding to the specimen DNA. A sharp signal is generated when probe DNA, bound to a specific target sequence in the specimen DNA, is visualized via fluorescent microscopy. Sequences as short as 1 kilobase can be detected in this manner, and the resolution between the sequences is usually in the range of 10-100 kilobases.

Large genomic changes, such as aneuploidy, deletions, and other chromosomal rearrangements, have long been associated with pregnancy loss, congenital abnormalities, and malignancy. These genomic changes are quantitative, unambiguous, and fundamental in the transition of normal cells to abnormal ones. Detection of these large genetic changes has an increasingly important role in determining patient diagnosis and care, including therapeutic selection. Vysis has developed two major product platforms that assess genomic changes at various levels of resolution. FISH techniques and the related technology of array-based comparative genomic hybridization (CGH) allow detection of gene sized or larger alterations in the genome. FISH is a robust DNA probe technology that can measure both balanced and unbalanced genomic changes on a cell-by-cell basis. In most instances, it is not dependent on metaphase chromosomes, and it is widely used in clinical diagnostics. Several modifications have taken place in FISH technology during recent years.

RNA diagnostics

Direct detection of RNA is desirable in some situations, particularly in the analysis of gene expression in human cells and tissues. RNA fragments are an alternative to diagnostics based on monoclonal antibodies (MAbs) and have the same specificity without the problems of maintaining hybridoma cells for producing antibody. Sequences of RNA can be screened for specific binding to a target. These binding stretches of RNA (aptamers) can be considered as synthesizable equivalents to MAb. Another important area of application is the detection of RNA viruses. The earliest test for this purpose was

Northern blot. RT-PCR is the most sensitive technique for mRNA detection and quantification currently available. Rapid deterioration of RNA is the most important impediment to RNA diagnostics. Several approaches have been used to reduce the rate at which RNA concentrations decline after the tissue is collected. Tests for RNA transcription are mostly aimed at RNA, with the exception of cycling probe technology (CPT) and Invader assay, which detects both RNA and DNA.

Cycling probe technology

Cycling probe technology (CPT) was developed by ID Biomedical and licensed to Takara Biomedical Group. It involves the introduction and multiplication of probes that are specific for the organisms being sought. Each probe is a sandwich of two short DNA segments attached to the two ends of an RNA segment. The probe attaches to a single strand of target DNA. Then the RNA strand is cut into two by RNase H, a naturally occurring enzyme. The two probe halves fall away, leaving the target strand free for another probe to attach. After about 45 minutes, the probe fragments are collected and can be detected by a color change in the sample following a routine immunology-based procedure. In contrast to PCR, CPT is isothermal with the probes floating in a sample solution along with RNase at a constant temperature. Probe amplification is linear and not exponential, thus eliminating carryover contamination, and also gives a quantitative assessment of viral or bacterial load. Because a single cleavage step is involved, the test is easy and cheap to produce and can be automated.

Linear RNA amplification

Incyte Corporation's Linear amplification technology is based on antisense RNA amplification and involves a series of enzymatic reactions resulting in T7-based linear amplification of RNA from small amounts of sample RNA. It can be applied to RNA obtained from small biopsies, mRNA-poor cells and tissues, primary cell culture and laser capture micro-dissection (LCM) samples. Unlike exponential amplification methods such as NASBA and RT-PCR, linear RNA amplification maintains relative ratios of the starting mRNA population (representational amplification). Linear RNA amplification technology is used to increase the levels of RNA expressed in cells to quantities that can be used for obtaining gene expression patterns on DNA microarrays and other related applications. This technology can be used for the development of novel diagnostics that identify gene expression patterns unique to particular diseases or disease subtypes.

Nucleic acid sequence-based amplification

Nucleic acid sequence-based amplification (NASBA) is the basis of the NucliSens system of Organon Teknika (now part of bioMerieux) and offers a simple and rapid alternative method for nucleic acid amplification. A description of the technology is available on the web site (http://www.nuclisens.com/). NucliSens represents a synergy of three key technologies – integrating isolation, molecular amplification and detection into an all-in-one system that is targeted at the sensitive and specific determination of nucleic acid sequences. NASBA technology is based on simultaneous enzymatic activity of reverse transcriptase, T7 RNA polymerase, and RNase in combination with two oligonucleotides. It depends on selective primer-template recognition to drive a cyclical, exponential amplification of the target sequence. NASBA has the following features:

- Unlike RT-PCR, NASBA is able to selectively amplify RNA sequences in a DNA background, since DNA strands are not melted out. There are no false positive signals due to dead bacteria.

- It can detect human mRNA sequences without the risk of DNA contamination; no intron flanking primers or Dnase approach is needed. This makes screening for gene expression in oncology or genetic diseases simple and easy.

- RNA amplification enables direct detection of RNA viruses such as HCV and retroviruses such as HIV.

- RNA targets permit the detection of live bacterial or viral activity following anti-bacterial/viral therapy.

- With RNA amplification, it is possible to observe the beginning of cancer cell proliferation through qualitative and quantitative determination of gene activity.

Introduction to biochip technology

Scientists and engineers are borrowing miniaturization, integration, and parallel-processing techniques from the computer industry to develop laboratory devices and procedures that will fit on a wafer or microchip. Biochip is a broad term indicating the use of microchip technology in molecular biology and can be defined as arrays of selected biomolecules immobilized on a surface. DNA microarray is a rapid method of sequencing and analyzing genes. An array is an orderly arrangement of samples. The sample spot sizes in microarray are usually less than 200 microns in diameter. It is comprised of DNA probes formatted on a microscale plus the instruments needed to handle samples (automated robotics), read the reporter molecules (scanners) and analyze the data (bioinformatic tools). Hybridization of RNA or DNA-derived samples on chips allows the monitoring of expression of mRNAs or the occurrence of polymorphisms in genomic DNA (Jain 2001).

In a DNA chip, an array of oligonucleotides or peptide nucleic acid probes is synthesized either in situ (on-chip) or by conventional synthesis followed by on-chip immobilization. The array is exposed to labeled sample DNA, hybridized, and the identity/abundance of complementary sequences is determined (Jain 2000). For practical purposes, the terms "DNA microarray" and "DNA chip" are used as synonyms although there are some technical differences as already indicated.

A microarray is a collection of miniaturized test sites arranged on a surface that permits many tests to be performed simultaneously, or in parallel, in order to achieve higher throughput. The average size of test sites in a microarray and the spacing between them defines the array's density. Higher density increases parallel processing throughput. In addition to increasing the throughput, higher density reduces the required volume for the sample being tested, and thereby lowers costs. Currently, the principal commercially available ways to produce microarrays include mechanical deposition, bead immobilization, inkjet printing and photolithography.

There are essentially three developments going on that aim to improve the presently available technique and to fulfill the requirements for second generation microarray systems: (1) new methods for label-free detection of the hybridization signals; (2) automatable flow-through systems; and (3) powerful data-processing software. Several biochip technologies will be mentioned later on in relation to nanobiotechnology.

Applications of biochips in diagnostics

Applications of biochip technologies in relation to molecular diagnostics are shown in Table 1-4.

Table 1-4: Applications of biochip technology in relation to molecular diagnostics.

Research applications
Molecular epidemiology
Study of gene expression in diseases
Rapid DNA sequencing
Design and stratification of clinical trials
Drug safety applications: pharmacogenetics and toxicogenomics
Genetic screening and detection of single nucleotide polymorphisms (SNPs)
Identification of pathogens and resistance in infections
Molecular oncology
Cancer prognosis
Cancer diagnosis
Cancer typing
Forensic identification: PCR on a chip
Detection of biological and chemical warfare agents
Public health: testing of water supply for microorganisms
Pharmacogenomics
Gene identification
Genetic mapping
Gene expression profiling
Integration of diagnosis and therapeutics

Proteomic technologies for molecular diagnostics

Although nucleic acid analysis of tissues by methods have been described earlier in this chapter is important, discovering the genetic sequence encoding a protein is not sufficient to predict the size or biological nature of a protein. Studies at the messenger RNA (mRNA) level can assess the expression profiles of transcripts but these analyses measure only the relative amount of an mRNA encoding a protein and not the actual amount of protein in a tissue. To address this area, several protein-based analysis technologies have been developed.

Proteomic technologies are considered to be a distinct group within molecular diagnostics and should not be confused with immunoassays although some proteomic technologies are antibody-based. These technologies are described in a special report on proteomics (Jain 2005a). The classical approaches in proteomics involve separating proteins by two-dimensional (2-D) gels and identify visualizing bands or spots. A modification of this technique is 2-D polyacrylamide gel electrophoresis (2-D PAGE). Protein can be detected by Western blot or fluorescence detection methods. The proteins are then analyzed and characterized using mass spectrometry and its modification – Matrix-Assisted Laser Desorption Mass Spectrometry (MALDI-MS). Other methods used include capillary electrophoresis, high performance liquid chromatography (HPLC) and electrospray ionization (ESI). The most comprehensive source of information on proteomics is found in protein sequence databases. Currently 2-D gel electrophoresis patterns are scanned into a computer and are then analyzed by computer algorithms that quantify the gel patterns according to whether they are obtained under normal or physiologically altered conditions.

MALDI-TOF Mass Spectrometry

Matrix Assisted Laser Desorption Ionization Time of Flight (MALDI-TOF) MS overcomes the rate-limiting step of the traditional mutation detection systems that require either radioactive, fluorescent or gel-based fragment detection and are limited in their speed and throughput. This approach separates and characterizes DNA and other molecules according to their mass: the fragment length does not limit charge ratio and the detection rate. Instead, MALDI-TOF works on the principle that each of the four DNA bases has its own signature mass: charge ratio and can, therefore, be identified as such. Each DNA sequence has its own unique mass and charge as determined by its base composition. Prepared samples form a matrix on a suitable carrier with light-absorbing crystals. The matrix is illuminated with a laser causing a small amount of sample to vaporize. An electrical pulse is applied to the flight tube upon launch and the 'time of flight' of the molecule is recorded with smaller molecules flying at a faster rate.

Detection by MS offers speed and high resolution. MALDI TOF MS can detect primer extension products, mass-tagged oligonucleotides, DNA created by restriction endonuclease cleavage, and genomic DNA. MALDI-TOF can be used to monitor nuclease selections of modified oligonucleotides with increased affinity for targets. Nuclease selections has been used for genotyping by treating DNA to be analyzed with oligonucleotide probes representing known genotypes and digesting probes that are not complementary to the DNA.

MALDI-TOF is much better at determining the masses of peptides than of DNA. A PCR product can be produced of any continuous region of coding sequence, which can then be used to encode an N-terminally tagged test peptide in a coupled in vitro transcription/translation reaction. The test peptide is purified using the tag, and its mass is measured by MALDI-TOF. Amino acid substitutions in peptides coded for by the breast cancer susceptibility gene BRCA1 have been identified using this method. The process can be multiplexed and is amenable to automation, providing an efficient, high-throughput means for mutation discovery and genetic profiling.

Differential Peptide Display

BioVisioN GmbH uses Differential Peptide Display (DPD) technology to analyse peptide patterns in biological sources such as body fluids, tissues, cells or cell-culture supernatant (Heine et al 2002). This enables the comparison of different patterns, e.g. of different groups of patients, in order to identify characteristic differences that correlate with the underlying metabolic or pathological events. DPD involves the extraction of peptides with a relative molecular mass of up to 20,000, concentration of this material, followed by HPLC-based separation into 96 fractions that are then submitted for mass spectrometric analysis using a MALDI-TOF MS. By recombining these 96 mass spectra, a comprehensive multi-dimensional fingerprint of peptides is obtained. It contains several thousand different signals, with each peptide's position characterized by its molecular mass and chromatographic behavior. Peptide patterns from different sets of samples are compared and differences that correlate with the investigated disease are detected. A comprehensive statistical analysis is used for evaluating detected differences. Promising candidates are sequenced, using tandem mass spectrometry (MS/MS) and Edman degradation.

DPD characterizes peptides with a relative molecular mass of between 800 and 20,000. This is particularly important in the analysis of plasma samples in a wide range of different diseases as many of the regulatory peptides and proteins that may be associated with the pathological events fall into these size fractions not normally detected in 2-DGE experiments.

Relation of molecular diagnostics to other technologies

Relation of molecular diagnostics to other technologies is shown in Figure 1-1. This is basis of some of the applications shown in the following section.

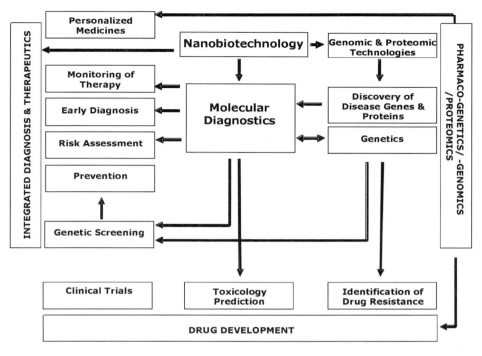

© Jain PharmaBiotech

Figure 1-1: Relation of nanobiotechnology to molecular diagnostics and other technologies

A confocal microscope image showing two colors of quantum dots – red and green – that are attached to different antibodies linking two unique structures on the surface of an infected cell. The color yellow indicates where the green and red dots are both present.

Applications of molecular diagnostics

Applications of molecular diagnostics are shown in Table 1-5.

Table 1-5: Applications of molecular diagnostics

Practice of medicine
As an aid to clinical diagnosis of various diseases
Diagnosis of disease susceptibility
Tissue typing in organ transplantation
Screening of blood transfusion
Combination of diagnosis and therapeutics
Development of personalized medicines
Forensic medicine for identification
Early and fast diagnosis of biowarfare agents
Use in biopharmaceutical industry
Use in drug discovery
Molecular toxicology
Pharmacogenomics
Pharmacogenetics
Gene therapy
DNA tagging for control and tracing of drug distribution channels
Detection of microbial contamination in biopharmaceutical manufacturing
Public health
Detection of food-borne pathogens
BSE detection
Testing for water supply safety
Molecular epidemiology

2. BASICS OF NANOBIOTECHNOLOGY

Abstract

This chapter describes the basics of nanotechnology, which is the popular term for the construction and utilization of functional structures with at least one characteristic dimension measured in nanometers - a nanometer is one billionth of a meter (10^{-9} m). Application of nanotechnology in relation to life sciences is considered a part of biotechnology and referred to as nanobiotechnology. Besides molecular diagnostics, related applications include drug discovery, drug delivery and eventually development of nanomedicine. The broad range of nanotechnologies relevant to molecular diagnostics range from devices to visualize biological structures on nanoscale such as atomic force microscopy to nanoparticles. Use of various nanomaterials for biolabeling is described. Research in life sciences is described as a foundation for molecular diagnostics and other healthcare applications of nanobiotechnology.

Introduction

Nanotechnology (Greek word nano means dwarf) is the creation and utilization of materials, devices, and systems through the control of matter on the nanometer-length scale, i.e., at the level of atoms, molecules, and supramolecular structures. It is the popular term for the construction and utilization of functional structures with at least one characteristic dimension measured in nanometers – a nanometer is one billionth of a meter (10^{-9} m). This is roughly four times the diameter of an individual atom and the bond between two individual atoms is 0.15 nm long. Proteins are 1 to 20 nanometers in size. The definition of 'small', another term used in relation to nanotechnology, depends on the application, but can range from 1 nm to 1 mm). Nano is not the smallest scale; further down the power of ten are angstrom (=0.1 nm), pico, femto, atto and zepto. By weight, the mass of a small virus is about 10 attograms. An attogram is one-thousandth of a femtogram, which is one-thousandth of a picogram, which is one-thousandth of a nanogram. Dimensions of various objects in nanoscale are shown in Table 2-1.

Table 2-1: Dimensions of various objects in nanoscale

Object	Dimension
Width of a hair	50,000 nm
Red blood cell	7,000 nm
Vesicle in a cell	200 nm
Bacterium	1,000 nm
Virus	100 nm
Exosomes (nanovesicles shed by dendritic cells)	65-100 nm
Width of DNA	2.5 nm
Ribosome	2-4 nm
A base pair in human genome	0.4 nm
Proteins	1-20 nm
Amino acid (e.g. tryptophan, the largest)	1.2 nm (longest measurement)
Aspirin molecule	1 nm
An individual atom	0.25 nm

Potential applications of nanotechnology include sensors, robotics, image processing, information technology, surface coatings, biomaterials, thin films, conducting polymers, photonics, liquid crystals, holography, virtual reality, surface engineering, smart materials micro-electronics, precision engineering and metrology.

Given the inherent nanoscale functional components of living cells, it was inevitable that nanotechnology will be applied in biotechnology giving rise to the term nanobiotechnology, which is focus of the report. The term "bionanotechnology" is being used synonymously with "nanobiotechnology" by some writers. As of 1 July 2005, "bionanotechnology" occurs only 16 times in MEDLINE search and appears only since 2004, whereas "nanobiotechnology" occurs 75 times and is used since 2000. Nanomaterials are at the leading edge of the rapidly developing field of nanotechnology; their unique size-dependent properties make these materials superior and indispensable in many areas of human activity (Salata 2004). A brief introduction will be given to basic nanotechnologies from physics and chemistry, which are now being integrated into molecular biology to advance the field of nanobiotechnology. The aim is to understand the biological processes to improve diagnosis and treatment of diseases. Technical achievements in nanotechnology are being applied to improve drug discovery, drug delivery and pharmaceutical manufacturing. Nanobiotechnologies and their applications are described in detail in a special report on this topic (Jain 2005b). A vast range of applications has spawned many new terms, which are defined as they are described in various chapters.

Landmarks in the evolution of nanobiotechnology

Historical landmarks in the evolution of nanobiotechnology are shown in Table 2-2.

Table 2-2: Historical landmarks in the evolution of nanotechnology and its diagnostic applications

Year	Landmark
1905	Einstein published a paper that estimated the diameter of a sugar molecular as about 1 nm
1931	Max Knoll and Ernst Ruska discover the electron microscope – enables subnanomolar imaging
1959	Nobel Laureate Richard Feynman gave a lecture entitled 'There's plenty of room at the bottom', at the annual meeting of the American Physical Society He outlined the principle of manipulating individual atoms using larger machines to manufacture increasingly smaller machines (Feynman 1992).
1974	Norio Tanaguchi of Japan coined the word "nanotechnology"
1979	Colloidal gold nanoparticles used as electron-dense probes in electron microscopy and immunocytochemistry (Batten and Hopkins 1979).
1984	The first description the term dendrimer and the method of preparation of poly(amidoamine) dendrimers (Tomalia et al 1985)
1985	Discovery of bucky balls (fullerenes) by Robert Curl, Richard Smalley and Harold Kroto, which led to the award of Nobel Prize for chemistry in 1996 (Smalley 1985; Curl et al 1997).
1987	Publication of the visionary book on nanotechnology potential "Engines of Creation" (Drexler 1987).
1988	Maturation of the field of supramolecular chemistry relevant to nanotechnology: construction of artificial molecules that interact with each other leading to award of Nobel prize (Lehn 1988).
1990	Atoms visualized by the scanning tunneling microscope discovered in 1980's at the IBM Zürich Laboratory (Zürich, Switzerland), which led to award of Nobel prize (Eigler and Schweizer 1990).
1991	Discovery of carbon nanotubes (Iijima et al 1992)
1997	Cancer targeting with nanoparticles coated with monoclonal antibodies (Douglas et al 1997)
1998	First use of nanocrystals as biological labels, which were shown to be superior to existing fluorphores (Bruchez et al 1998)
2000	Nanotechnology Initiative announced in the US (Roco 2000). The worldwide emergence of nanoscale science and engineering.
2003	The US Senate passed the Nanotechnology Research & Development Act making the National Nanotechnology Initiative into law and authorized \$3.7 billion over the next 4 years for the program

© JainPharmaBiotech

Classification of nanobiotechnologies

It is not easy to classify the vast range of nanobiotechnologies. Some just represent motion on a nanoscale but most of them are based on nanoscale structures, which come in a variety of shapes and sizes. A few occur in nature but most are engineered. The word nano is prefixed to just about anything that deals with nanoscale. It is not just biotechnology but many other disciplines such as nanophysics, nanobiology, etc. A simplified classification of basic nanobiotechnologies is shown in Table 2-3. Some technologies such as nanoarrays and nanochips are further developments.

Table 2-3: Classification of basic nanobiotechnologies

Visualization and manipulation at nanoscale
Atomic force microscopy
Scanning probe microscopy
Nanomanipulation
Surface plasmon resonance
Femtosecond laser systems
Nanoscale motion
Cantilevers
Nanoparticles
Quantum dots
Nanocrystals
Lipoparticles
Magnetic nanoparticles
Polymer nanoparticles
Nanofibers
Nanowires
Carbon nanofibers
Dendrimers
Polypropylenimine dendrimers
Composite nanostructures
Nanoemulsions
Nanolipisomes
Nanocapsules enclosing other substances
Nanoshells
Nanovesicles
Cochleates
Nanoconduits
Nanotubes
Nanopipettes
Nanoneedles
Nanochannels
Nanopores
Nanofluidics
Nanostructured silicon

We are learning from nature in nanotechnology, particularly nanobiotechnology. Nature constructs complex, efficient self-organizing and self-regulating molecular machinery and systems for all processes in living organisms. Some of the examples of this are described in Chapter 3. Nature has made highly precise and functional nanostructures for billions of years: DNA, proteins, membranes, etc, but it is only since the 1980's that man has been able to manufacture such precise synthetic nanostructures at will. Nanostructures are made from thousands of atoms that are precisely defined in space. They have an unlimited number of compositions, sizes, shapes and most importantly, functionality.

Technologies for visualization of biological structures at nanoscale

Atomic force microscopy

Basic AFM operation

In its most basic form, atomic force microscopy (AFM) images topography by precisely scanning a probe across the sample to "feel" the contours of the surface. The interaction between the needle and the surface is measured and an image is reconstructed from the data collected in this manner. With AFM, it is possible it is possible to reach an extremely high resolution. Because it can be applied under standard conditions in an aqueous environment, any significant perturbation of the sample can be avoided. In contrast to light microscopy and scanning electron microscopy, AFM provides the most optimal means to investigate the surface structures in three dimensions, with resolutions as high as 0.1-0.2 nm.

A key element of the AFM is its microscopic force sensor, or cantilever. The cantilever is usually formed by one or more beams of silicon or silicon nitride that is 100 to 500 microns long and about 0.5 to 5 microns thick. Mounted on the end of the cantilever is a sharp tip that is used to sense a force between the sample and tip. For normal topographic imaging, the probe tip is brought into continuous or intermittent contact with the sample and raster-scanned over the surface.

Advantages of AFM

In addition to its superior resolution and routine three-dimensional measurement capability, AFM offers several other clear advantages over traditional microscopy techniques. For example, scanning and transmission electron microscopy (SEM, TEM) image biologically inactive, dehydrated samples and generally require extensive sample preparation such as staining or metal coating. AFM eliminates these requirements and, in many cases, allows direct observation of native specimens and ongoing processes under native or near-native conditions.

Further adding to its uniqueness, the AFM can directly measure nanoscale interactive forces, e.g., ligand-receptor binding. Samples can be examined in ambient air or biological fluids without the cost and inconvenience of vacuum equipment. Sample preparation is minimal and allows the use of standard techniques for optical microscopy. The MultiMode AFM provides maximal resolution while the BioScope AFM integrates the best of optical and atomic force microscopy to help life scientists explore new frontiers.

The ability of the atomic force microscope (AFM) to create three-dimensional micrographs with resolution down to the nanometer and Angstrom scales has made it an essential tool for imaging surfaces in applications ranging from semiconductor processing to cell biology. In addition to this topographical imaging, however, the AFM can also probe nanomechanical and other fundamental properties of sample surfaces, including their local adhesive or elastic (compliance) properties.

Microscopic adhesion affects a huge variety of events, from the behavior of paints and glues, ceramics and composite materials, to DNA replication and the action of drugs in the human body. Elastic properties are similarly important, often affecting the structural and dynamic behavior of systems from composite materials to blood cells. AFM offers a new tool to study these important parameters on the micron to nanometer scale using a technique that measures forces on the AFM probe tip as it approaches and retracts from a surface.

Magnetic resonance force microscopy

IBM has been working over a decade to develop nanoscale magnetic resonance imaging technology called magnetic resonance force microscopy (MRFM). The company claimed a breakthrough in nanoscale magnetic resonance imaging by directly detecting for the first time a faint magnetic signal from single electrons buried inside solid samples. The development represents a major milestone in the creation of a microscope that can make three-dimensional images of molecules with atomic resolution. Such a device could have a major impact on the study of materials, ranging from proteins and pharmaceuticals to integrated circuits for which a detailed understanding of the atomic structure is essential.

Knowing the exact location of specific atoms within tiny nano-electronic structures, for example, could enhance circuit and chip designers' insight into their manufacture and performance, according to IBM. The ability to image the detailed atomic structure of proteins directly would also aid the development of new drugs. This new capability should ultimately lead to fundamental advances in nanotechnology and biology.

The central feature of MRFM is a silicon 'micro-cantilever' that looks like a miniature diving board and is 1,000 times thinner than a human hair. It vibrates at a frequency of about 5,000 times a second, and a tiny but powerful magnetic particle attached to the tip attracts or repels individual electrons. Such technology aims to boost magnetic resonance imaging sensitivity by some 10 million times compared to the medical devices currently used to visualize organs in the human body. The magnetic sensors are crucial for high resolution magnetic force microscopy. They are coated with suitably layered materials.

Scanning probe microscopy

The scanning probe microscope (SPM) system is emerging as an increasingly important tool for non-intrusive interrogation of biomolecular systems in vitro. Its particular merit is that it retains complete functionality in a biocompatible fluid environment and can track the dynamics of cellular and molecular processes in real time and real space at nm resolution, as an imaging tool, and with pN force-sensing/imposing resolution, as an interaction tool (Myhra 2004). The capability may have relevance as a test bed for monitoring cellular response to environmental stimuli and pharmaceutical intervention. The better-known recent contributions of SPM are towards explanatory and predictive descriptions of biomolecular interactions at surfaces and interfaces, and there are some recent attempts to reconfigure the SPM platform for demonstration of novel bio-device applications.

SPM enables high resolution without any of the drawbacks of electron microscopy, which can damage sensitive molecules by electrons. SPM enables investigation of biomolecules in fluid environments under physiological conditions and is useful for study of biology on nanoscale.

Multiple single-molecule fluorescence microscopy

Fitting the image of a single molecule to the point spread function of an optical system greatly improves the precision with which single molecules can be located. In nanometer-localized multiple single-molecule (NALMS) fluorescence microscopy, short duplex DNA strands are used as nanoscale "rulers" for validation (Qu et al 2004). Nanometer accuracy was demonstrated for 2-5 single molecules within a diffraction-limited area. NALMS microscopy will greatly facilitate single-molecule study of biological systems because it covers the gap between fluorescence resonance energy transfer-based (<10 nm) and diffraction-limited microscopy (>100 nm) measurements of the distance between two fluorophores. NALMS microscopy has been applied to DNA mapping with <10-nm resolution.

Nanoparticle characterization by Halo™ LM10 technology

Halo™ LM10 (NanoSight Ltd) is based on the laser illumination of a specially designed optical element on to which sample is simply placed manually or allowed to flow across the surface. This is the first nanoparticle characterization tool, specifically designed for liquid phase sizing of individual nanoparticles, with the use of a conventional light microscope. Particles as small as 20 nm have been successfully visualized by this method, each particle being seen as an individual point of light moving under Brownian motion within the liquid. The intensity of light scattered by a particle varies as the 6th power of its radius. By doubling the diameter of the particle, 64-fold more light is scattered by the particle. This has significant implications for the early and simple detection of aggregation, flocculation and dimerization of particulates at the nanometer scale.

Use of a shorter wavelength laser source capable of exciting fluorescent labels enables specific components within the sample to be distinguished from non-specific background particles. The image can be analyzed by suitable software allowing changes in individual particle position to be followed furnishing real time information about particle diffusion and particle-to-particle interactions. In the fluorescence mode, correlation techniques can be used to derive information by use of the technique known as fluorescence correlation spectroscopy. Halo™ LM10 is supported by Halo™ GS10 software.

The laser source need only be a few mW in power and can be delivered to the optical device via fibreoptic connection or the laser diode can be coupled directly to the edge of the optical element. The optical element can be manufactured in optical quality plastic or in glass or silica. The optical element need only be a few mm square and 2-5 mm in depth.

Larger volumes of sample containing dilute concentrations of particles of interest can be analyzed by being configured within a flow cell. Fabrication of the optical element is by industry standard metal coating techniques such as those found in the electronics and optical devices industries. Applications relevant to molecular diagnostics are:

- Detection of viral particles: diagnosis of viral diseases, e.g. cerebrospinal fluid

- DNA analysis

- Mycoplasma detection in animal cell culture

- Cancer cell detection, e.g., metastases

Nanoscale scanning electron microscopy

Three-dimensional (3D) structural information is important in biological research. Excellent methods are available to obtain structures of molecules at atomic, organelles at electron microscopic, and of tissue at light-microscopic resolution. However, there is a need to reconstruct 3D tissue structure with a nanoscale resolution to identify small organelles such as synaptic vesicles. Such 3D data are essential to understand cellular networks that need to be completely reconstructed throughout a substantial spatial volume, particularly in the nervous system. Datasets meeting these requirements can be obtained by automated block-face imaging combined with serial sectioning inside the chamber of a SEM (Denk and Horstmann 2004). Backscattering contrast is used to visualize the heavy-metal staining of tissue prepared using techniques that are routine for TEM. The resolution is sufficient to trace even the thinnest axons and to identify synapses. Stacks of several hundred sections, 50-70 nm thick, have been obtained at a lateral position jitter of typically under 10 nm. This opens up the possibility of automatically obtaining the electron-microscope-level 3D datasets needed to completely reconstruct the neuronal circuits.

Optical imaging with a silver superlens

A superlens has been created that can overcome a limitation in physics that has historically constrained the resolution of optical images (Fang et al 2005). Using a thin film of silver as the lens and ultraviolet light, images of an array of nanowires can be recorded at a resolution of about 60 nm, whereas current optical microscopes can only make out details down to 400 nm. This work has a far reaching impact on the development of detailed biomedical imaging. With current optical microscopes, scientists can only make out relatively large structures within a cell, such as its nucleus and mitochondria. With a superlens, optical microscopes could reveal the movements of individual proteins traveling along the microtubules that make up a cell's skeleton. SEM and AFM are now used to capture detail down to a few nanometers. However, such microscopes create images by scanning objects point by point, which means they are typically limited to non-living samples, and image capture times can take up to several minutes. Optical microscopes can capture an entire frame with a single snapshot in a fraction of a second, opening up nanoscale imaging to living materials, which can help biologists better understand cell structure and function in real time, and ultimately help in the development of new drugs to treat human diseases.

Fluorescence resonance energy transfer

Fluorescence resonance energy transfer (FRET) is a process by which energy that would normally be emitted as a photon from an excited fluorophore can be directly transferred to a second fluorophore to excite one of its electrons. This, on decay, then generates an even longer wavelength photon. The extent of FRET is critically dependent on the distance between the two fluorophores as well as their spectral overlap. Thus FRET is a powerful reporter of the separation of the two fluorophores. FRET is a simple but effective tool for measurements of protein-protein interactions. It is one of the few techniques that are capable of giving dynamic information about the nanometer-range proximity between molecules, as opposed to simply the subcellular co-localization that is provided by fluorescence microscopy.

Nanolasers

The nanolasers were developed by growing semiconductor nanowires. The linewidths, wavelengths, and power dependence of the nanowire emission characterize the nanowires as active optical cavities. Current leading solid-state lasers, often made of gallium arsenide or gallium nitride, are made of multilayer thin films and measure several micrometers in size. The nanowire laser is 1,000 times smaller, allowing localized optical illumination. It can be tuned to emit light of different wavelengths from the infrared to the deep ultraviolet by simply changing the diameter or composition of the nanowire.

One of the smallest lasers ever made, nanowire nanolaser, is too small to be seen even with the aid of the most powerful optical microscope.

The nanowire nanolasers are pure crystals of zinc oxide that grow vertically in aligned arrays like the bristles on a brush. These crystal nanowires range from 2-10 microns in length, depending upon how long the growth process was allowed to proceed. The nanowire nanolaser emits flashes of ultraviolet light, measures just less than 100 nm. The individual ZnO nanowires have uniform diameters ranging from 10-300 nm. Under optical excitation, each individual ZnO nanowire serves as a Fabry-Perot optical cavity, and together they form a highly ordered nanowire ultraviolet laser array (Yan et al 2003).

It is the small area of illumination that holds near-term potential for the nanolaser. Near-term products could include ultrahigh resolution photolithography for next-generation microchips, as well as laser-powered biochips. Other potential applications for the nanolaser include high-density information storage, high-definition displays, photonics, optocommunications and chemical analysis on microchips. Nanolasers have also been used to study very small biological structures.

Nanoparticles

Nanoparticles can be made of different materials, e.g., gold. A nanoparticle contains tens to thousands of atoms and exists in a realm that straddles the quantum and the Newtonian. At those sizes every particle has new properties that change depending on its size. As matter is shrunk to nanoscale, electronic and other properties change radically. Nanoparticles may contain unusual forms of structural disorder that can significantly modify materials properties and thus cannot solely be considered as small pieces of bulk material (Gilbert et al 2004). Two nanoparticles, both made of pure gold, can exhibit markedly different behavior – different melting temperature, different electrical conductivity, different color – if one is larger than the other. That creates a new way to control the properties of materials. Instead of changing composition, one can change size. Some applications of nanoparticles take advantage of the fact that more surface area is exposed when material is broken down to smaller sizes. For magnetic nanoparticles, the lack of blemishes produces magnetic fields remarkably strong considering the size of the particles. Nanoparticles are also so small that in most of them, the atoms line up in perfect crystals without a single blemish.

Zinc sulfide nanoparticles a mere 10 atoms across have a disordered crystal structure that puts them under constant strain, increasing the stiffness of the particles and probably affecting other properties, such as strength and elasticity. In similar semiconducting nanoparticles, such as those made of cadmium selenide, slight differences in size lead to absorption and emission of different wavelengths of light, making them useful as fluorescent tracers. The dominant cause of such properties is quantum mechanical confinement of the electrons in a small package. But the disordered crystal structure now found in nanoparticles could affect light absorption and emission also. X-ray diffraction of single nanoparticles is not yet possible and other methods are used to analyze X-ray diffraction images of nanoparticles so as to separate the effects of size from those of disordered structure. Some nanoparticles that are relevant to molecular diagnostics will be described briefly in this chapter. The best known of these are quantum dots.

Quantum dots

Quantum dots (QDs) are nanoscale crystals of semiconductor material that glow, or fluoresce when excited by a light source such as a laser. QD nanocrystals of cadmium selenide 200-10,000 atoms wide, coated with zinc sulfide. The size of the QD determines the frequency of light emitted when irradiated with low energy light. The QDs were initially found to be unstable and difficult to use in solution. Work at Indiana University (Bloomington, IN) showed that embedding the dots in pores of a latex bead made them more stable. Multicolor optical coding for biological assays has been achieved by embedding different-sized QDs into polymeric microbeads at precisely controlled ratios. Their novel optical properties (e.g., size-tunable emission and simultaneous excitation) render these highly luminescent QDs ideal fluorophores for wavelength-and-intensity multiplexing. The use of 10 intensity levels and six colors could theoretically code one million nucleic acid or protein sequences. Imaging and spectroscopic measurements indicate that the QD-tagged beads are highly uniform and reproducible, yielding bead identification accuracies as high as 99.99% under favorable conditions. DNA hybridization studies demonstrate that the coding and target signals can be simultaneously read at the single-bead level. This spectral coding technology is expected to open new opportunities in gene expression studies, high-throughput screening, and medical diagnostics.

Latex beads filled with several colors of nanoscale semiconductor QDs can serve as unique labels for any number of different probes. When exposed to light, the beads identify themselves and their linked probes by emitting light in a distinct spectrum of colors – a sort of spectral bar code. The shape and size of quantum dots can be tailored to fluoresce specific colors. Current dyes used for lighting up protein and DNA fade quickly, but quantum dots could allow tracking of biological reactions in living cells for days or longer.

A scalable method has been reported for controlled synthesis of luminescent QDs using microemulsion-gas contacting at room temperature (Karanikolos et al 2004). The technique exploits the dispersed phase of a microemulsion to form numerous identical nanoreactors. In this approach, ZnSe quantum dots are synthesized by reacting hydrogen selenide gas with diethylzinc dissolved in the heptane nanodroplets of a microemulsion formed by self-assembly of a poly(ethylene oxide)-poly(propylene oxide)-poly(ethylene oxide) amphiphilic block copolymer in formamide. A single nanocrystal is grown in each nanodroplet, thus allowing good control of particle size by manipulation of the initial diethylzinc concentration in the heptane. The ZnSe nanocrystals exhibit size-dependent luminescence and excellent photostability. The particle-loaded emulsions are very stable in storage for months.

QDs can also be placed in a strong magnetic field, which gives an electron on the dot two allowed energy states separated by an energy gap that depends on the strength of the field. The electron can jump the gap by absorbing a photon of precisely that energy, which can be tuned, by altering the field, to correspond with the energy of a far-infrared photon. Once it is excited by absorption of a photon, the electron can leap onto the terminal of a single-electron transistor, where it 'throws the switch' and is detected. One device can register an incoming signal of just one photon every ten seconds on an area of 0.1 square millimeters, making it ten thousand times more sensitive than previous far-infrared light detectors (Komiyama et al 2000). QDs are used in molecular diagnostics.

Gold nanoparticles

DNA molecules are attached to gold nanoparticles, which tangle with other specially designed pieces of DNA into clumps that appear blue. The presence of lead causes the connecting DNA to fall apart. That cuts loose the individual gold nanoparticles and changes the color from blue to red. Gold nanoparticles are also used as a connecting point to build biosensors for detection of disease. A common technique for a diagnostic test consists of an antibody attached to a fluorescent molecule. When the antibody attaches to a protein associated with the disease, the fluorescent molecule lights up under ultraviolet light. Instead of a fluorescent molecule, a gold nanoparticle can be attached to the antibody and other molecules such as DNA can be added to the nanoparticle to produce bar codes. Because many copies of the antibodies and DNA can be attached to a single nanoparticle, this approach is much more sensitive and accurate than the fluorescent-molecule tests used currently.

43

Biomedical applications of self-assembly of nanoparticles

Researchers at Sandia National Laboratories and the University of New Mexico have perfected a commercially feasible way for orderly arrays of nanoparticles to self-assemble, each insulated from the others by silicon dioxide. The technique will not only enable new devices but could also solve one of the longest-standing problems with nanoparticles: forming orderly connections between the microscale and the nanoscale. The self-assembly technique prevents nanoparticles from clumping plus insulated them from each other with silicon dioxide. By spin-coating precisely controlled thicknesses of silicon dioxide with embedded nanoparticles, the researchers hope to reduce to nanoscale the applications that until now have resisted downsizing. For example, the nanoparticles could be formed into thin films for nanoscale lasers, whose frequency depends on the nanoparticles' size.

The patented process created at Sandia uses an organic surfactant layer that ordinarily makes it difficult to process nanoparticles. Acting like a kind of grease, the patented approach scrubs the surfactants off the nanoparticles with an ozone compound and instead embeds them in oxide. In the two-step process, first a detergent solution is mixed with the nanoparticles, scrubbing off the grease and thereby making them water-soluble. In the second step, silica is introduced into the solution causing the nanoparticles to embed themselves into a silicon dioxide lattice when the compound solidifies. The three-dimensional films and solids created with the process are stable indefinitely and can have application-specific ligands attached for biomedical devices. Even nanoparticles of different types could be combined to create specialized nanomolecules.

This approach should ease the transition from the micron-sized connections on currently available commercial chips to the orders-of-magnitude denser nanoscale structures. By using self-assembly techniques compatible with standard microelectronic processing, huge gaps in scale can be bridged by integrating nanocrystal arrays into standard silicon chips. The nanoparticles embedded in silicon dioxide could become a massive number of stored charge cells. In the test material, the researchers demonstrated a kind of choreographed transmission among nanoparticles called a "Coulomb blockade." At low voltages no current passes, because each nanoparticle is separated from adjacent ones by a layer of silicon dioxide several nanometers thick. But at high voltages, current jumped by the cube of the voltage.

In addition, because nanoparticles typically range from 1-10 nm in diameter, their electrical properties are dominated by quantum confinement effects. Coulomb interactions in nanoparticles form excitons (electron-hole pairs) when they are pumped with optical energy from a laser. The distance between the electron and hole is called the Bohr radius of the exciton and the resultant energized nanoparticle is called a quantum dot. By merely changing the size of a quantum dot, one can get different frequencies of emission upon pumping by a laser. For example, one can get them to emit light could make them useful adjuncts to molecules that are being created to bind to cancer cells. Sandia Laboratories has applied for a patent for identifying cancer cells early with such fluorescent markers.

Superparamagnetic iron oxide nanoparticles

Superparamagnetic iron oxide nanoparticles (SPION) with appropriate surface chemistry have been widely used experimentally for numerous in vivo applications such as magnetic resonance imaging (MRI) contrast enhancement, tissue repair, immunoassay, detoxification of biological fluids, hyperthermia, drug delivery and in cell separation, etc. These applications require that these nanoparticles have high magnetization values and size smaller than 100 nm with overall narrow particle size distribution, so that the particles have uniform physical and chemical properties. In addition, these applications need special surface coating of the magnetic particles, which has to be not only nontoxic and biocompatible but also allow a targetable delivery with particle localization in a specific area. Nature of surface coatings of the nanoparticles determines not only the overall size of the colloid but also plays a significant role in biokinetics and biodistribution of nanoparticles in the body. Magnetic nanoparticles can bind to drugs, proteins, enzymes, antibodies, or nucleotides and can be directed to an organ, tissue, or tumor using an external magnetic field or can be heated in alternating magnetic fields for use in hyperthermia (Gupta and Gupta 2005).

Magnetic labeling of cells provides the ability to monitor their temporal spatial migration in vivo by MRI. Various methods have been used to magnetically label cells using SPIONs. Magnetic tagging of stem cells and other mammalian cells has the potential for guiding future cell-based therapies in humans and for the evaluation of cellular-based treatment effects in disease models.

Use of superparamagnetic nanoparticles for study of living cells

Technologies to assess the molecular targets of biomolecules in living cells are lacking. A new technology called magnetism-based interaction capture (MAGIC) has been developed that identifies molecular targets on the basis of induced movement of superparamagnetic nanoparticles (MNP) inside living cells (Won et al 2005). The scientists painted intracellular proteins with fluorescent materials and inserted magnetic nanoparticles-embedded drugs into the cell. These nanoprobes captured the small molecule's labeled target protein and were translocated in a direction specified by the magnetic field. Use of MAGIC in genome-wide expression screening identified multiple protein targets of a drug. MAGIC was also used to monitor signal-dependent modification and multiple interactions of proteins. It was also shown that internalized MNPs could be moved inside cells by an external magnetic field, using a luminescent nanocrystal quantum dot, which does not exhibit magnetism, as a control. The MNPs not only responded to application of the magnetic field but they also rapidly dispersed when the magnetic field was removed and reassembled on reapplication of the magnetic field. MAGIC can be useful in the development of diagnostics and biosensors. Its ultimate use would be for the analysis of interactions inside living cells of patients.

Fluorescent nanoparticles

Fluorescent nanoparticles can be used as labels for immunometric assay of C-reactive protein (CRP) using two-photon excitation assay technology (Koskinen et al 2004). This new assay technique enables multiplexed, separation-free bioaffinity assays from microvolumes with high sensitivity. The assay of CRP was optimized for assessment of CRP baseline levels using a nanoparticulate fluorescent reporter, 75nm in diameter, and the assay performance was compared to that of CRP assay based on a molecular reporter of the same fluorophore core. The results show that using fluorescent nanoparticles as the reporter provides two orders of magnitude better sensitivity than using the molecular label, while no difference between precision profiles of the different assay types was found. The new assay method was applied for assessment of baseline levels of CRP in sera of apparently healthy individuals.

Scientists at the Institut für Materialforschung at the Forschungszentrum (Karlsruhe, Germany) are using microwave plasma technique to develop fluorescent nanoparticles. In a second reaction, a layer of organic dye is deposited and the final step is an outer cover of polymer, which protects the nanoparticles from exposure to environments. Each layer has characteristic properties. The size of the particles varies and these are being investigated for applications in molecular diagnostics.

Nanoshells

Nanoshells are are ball-shaped structures about the size of a virus or 1/20th of a RBC. They consist of a core of non-conducting glass that is covered by a metallic shell, typically either gold or silver. Nanoshells possess highly favorable optical and chemical properties for biomedical imaging and therapeutic applications. By varying the relative the dimensions of the core and the shell, the optical resonance of these nanoparticles can be precisely and systematically varied over a broad region ranging from the near-UV to the mid-infrared. This range includes the near-infrared (NIR) wavelength region where tissue transmissibility peaks. In addition to spectral tunability, nanoshells offer other advantages over conventional organic dyes including improved optical properties and reduced susceptibility to chemical/thermal denaturation. Furthermore, the same conjugation protocols used to bind biomolecules to gold colloid are easily modified for nanoshells. The core/shell ratio and overall size of a gold nanoshell influences its scattering and absorption properties. Nanoshell-based diagnostic and therapeutic approaches are in development including the development of nanoshell bioconjugates for molecular imaging, the use of scattering nanoshells as contrast agents for optical coherence tomography.

Gold Nanoshells (Spectra Biosciences) possess physical properties similar to gold colloid, in particular a strong optical absorption due to the collective electronic response of the metal to light. The optical absorption of gold colloid yields a brilliant red color, which has been of considerable utility in consumer-related medical products such as home pregnancy tests. In contrast, the optical response of gold Nanoshells depends dramatically on the relative sizes of the nanoparticle core and the thickness of the gold shell. By varying the relative core and shell thickness, the color of gold Nanoshells can be varied across a broad range of the optical spectrum that spans the visible and the near-infra red spectral regions. Gold Nanoshells can be made either to absorb or scatter light preferentially by varying the size of the particle relative to the wavelength of the light at their optical resonance.

Carbon nanotubes

Carbon nanotubes are rolled-up sheets of carbon atoms that appear naturally in soot, and are central to many nanotechnology projects. These nanotubes can go down in diameter to 1 nm, are stronger than any material in the universe and can be any length. Minuscule webs of connected carbon nanotubes can be grown. Single-wall carbon nanotubes can be used as probes for AFMs that can image individual molecules in both wet and dry environments. Nanotubes could be used as biosensors. Fabricating structures on the nanoscale, however, is a formidable challenge because current methods to controllably synthesize nanotubes limit their complexity. A technique has been devised to create multiply connected and hierarchically branched nanopores inside of anodic aluminum oxide templates (Meng et al 2005). This method can produce combinations of Y shapes and multiple branches, yielding a wealth of new architectures that could be used to design nanoscale biomaterials. Applications of carbon nanotubes relevant to molecular diagnostics are:

- It is possible to insert DNA into a carbon nanotube. Devices based on the DNA-nanotube combination could eventually be used to sequence DNA electronically.

- Carbon nanotubes can be used as tips for AFM

- Carbon nanotubes can be used in biosensors

- Carbon nanotubes can be used as biological imaging agents

The uptake of single-walled carbon nanotubes (SWNTs) into macrophage-like cells has been studied using the nanotubes' intrinsic near-infrared fluorescence (Cherukuri et al 2004). Nanotube uptake appears to occur through phagocytosis. There were no adverse effects on the cells and the nanotubes retained their unique optical properties. The new findings suggest that SWNTs might be valuable biological imaging agents, in part because SWNTs fluoresce in the near-infrared portion of the spectrum, at wavelengths not normally emitted by biological tissues. This may allow light from even a handful of nanotubes to be selectively detected from within the body. Although long term studies on toxicity and biodistributions must be completed before nanotubes can be used in medical tests, the new findings indicate nanotubes could soon be useful as imaging markers in laboratory in vitro studies, particularly in cases where the bleaching, toxicity and degradation of more traditional markers are problematic.

Nanowires

The manipulation of photons in structures smaller than the wavelength of light is central to the development of nanoscale integrated photonic systems for computing, communications, and sensing. Scientists at the Lawrence Berkeley National Laboratory (Berkeley, CA) have assembled small groups of freestanding, chemically synthesized nanoribbons and nanowires into model structures that illustrate how light is exchanged between subwavelength cavities made of three different semiconductors (Sirbuly et al 2005). With simple coupling schemes, lasing nanowires can launch coherent pulses of light through ribbon waveguides that are up to a millimeter in length. Also, interwire coupling losses are low enough to allow light to propagate across several right-angle bends in a grid of crossed ribbons. Nanoribbons function efficiently as waveguides in liquid media and provide a unique means for probing molecules in solution or in proximity to the waveguide surface. These results lay the groundwork for photonic devices based on assemblies of active and passive nanowire elements. There are potential applications of nanowire waveguides in microfluidics and biology. Some Nanowire-based nanobiosensors are in development.

Dendrimers

Dendrimers (dendri - tree, mer - branch) are a novel class of three-dimensional nanoscale, core-shell structures that can be precisely synthesized for a wide range of applications. Specialized chemistry techniques allow for precise control over the physical and chemical properties of the dendrimers. They are constructed generation by generation in a series of controlled steps that increase the number of small branching molecules around a central core molecule. Up to ten generations can be incorporated into a single dendrimer molecule. The final generation of molecules added to the growing structure makes up the polyvalent surface of the dendrimer (see Figure 2-1). The core, branching and surface molecules are chosen to give desired properties and functions.

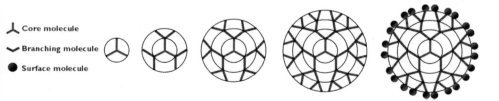

Source: Starpharma Holding Ltd, by permission

Figure 2-1: The core, branching and surface molecules of dendrimers

As a result of their unique architecture and construction, dendrimers possess inherently valuable physical, chemical and biological properties. These include:

- Precise architecture, size and shape control. Dendrimers branch out in a highly predictable fashion to form amplified three-dimensional structures with highly ordered architectures.

- High uniformity and purity. The proprietary step-wise synthetic process used produces dendrimers with highly uniform sizes (monodispersity) possessing precisely defined surface functionality and very low impurity levels.

- High loading capacity. Internal cavities intrinsic to dendrimer structures can be used to carry and store a wide range of metals, organic, or inorganic molecules.

- High shear resistance. Through their three-dimensional structure dendrimers have a high resistance to shear forces and solution conditions.

- Low toxicity. Most dendrimer systems display very low cytotoxicity levels.

- Low immunogenicity when injected or used topically.

The surface properties of dendrimers may be manipulated by the use of appropriate 'capping' reagents on the outermost generation. In this way dendrimers can be readily decorated to yield a novel range of functional properties including flexible binding properties. By using appropriate capping groups on the dendrimer exterior, dendrimers can be designed to exhibit strong affinity for specific targets.

While the potential applications of dendrimers are unlimited, some of their current uses relevant to molecular diagnostics include biosensors and imaging contrast agents.

Cantilevers

Cantilevers (Concentris) transform a chemical reaction into a mechanical motion on the nanometer scale. Measurements of a cantilever are: length 500 μm, width 100 μm, thickness 25-500 μm and deflection 10 nm. This motion can be measured directly by deflecting a light beam from the cantilever surface. Concentris uses an array of parallel VCSELs (Vertical Cavity Surface Emitting Lasers) as stable, robust and proven light source. A state-of-the-art position sensitive detector is employed as detection device.

The static mode is used to obtain information regarding the presence of certain target molecules in the sample substance. The surface stress caused by the adsorption of these molecules results in minute deflections of the cantilever. This deflection directly correlates with the concentration of the target substance. The dynamic mode allows quantitative analysis of mass loads in the sub-picogram area. As molecules get adsorbed, minimal shifts in the resonance frequency of an oscillating cantilever can be measured and associated to reference data of the target substance. Both modes can also be operated simultaneously.

The controlled deposition of functional layers is the key to converting nanomechanical cantilevers into chemical or biochemical sensors. Inkjet printing as a rapid and general method to coat cantilever arrays efficiently with various sensor layers (Bietsch et al 2004). Self-assembled monolayers of alkanethiols are deposited on selected Au-coated cantilevers and rendered them sensitive to ion concentrations or pH in liquids. The detection of gene fragments is achieved with cantilever sensors coated with thiol-linked single-stranded DNA oligomers on Au. A selective etch protocol proves the uniformity of the monolayer coatings at a microscopic level. A chemical gas sensor is fabricated by printing thin layers of different polymers from dilute solutions onto cantilevers. The inkjet method is easy to use, faster and more versatile than coating via microcapillaries or the use of pipettes. In addition, it is scalable to large arrays and can coat arbitrary structures in non-contact.

The diagnostic applications of cantilever technology, Cantosens (Concentris) are :

- Parallel and label-free detection of disease markers, e.g. serum proteins or autoantibodies.

- Fast, label-free recognition of specific DNA sequences (SNPs, oncogenes, genotyping)

- Detection of microorganisms and antimicrobial susceptibility

- Detection of trace contaminations in food, e.g. antibiotics, hormones, pesticides

- Environmental monitoring: detection of pesticides, air pollutants

- Water analysis

Surface plasmon resonance

Surface plasmon resonance (SPR) is an optical-electrical phenomenon involving the interaction of light with the electrons of a metal. The optical-electronic basis of SPR is the transfer of the energy carried by photons of light to a group of electrons (a plasmon) at the surface of a metal. Light is coupled into the surface plasmon by means of either a prism or a grating on the metal surface. Depending on the thickness of a molecular layer at the metal surface, the SPR phenomenon results in a graded reduction in intensity of the reflected light. Biomedical applications take advantage of the exquisite sensitivity of SPR to the refractive index of the medium next to the metal surface, which makes it possible to measure accurately the adsorption of molecules on the metal surface and their eventual interactions with specific ligands. Applications of this technique include the following:

- Measurement in real-time of the kinetics of ligand-receptor interactions

- Screening of lead compounds in the pharmaceutical industry

- Measurement of DNA hybridization

- Enzyme-substrate interactions

- Polyclonal antibody characterization

- Protein conformation studies

- Label-free immunoassays.

Nanostamping

The technology uses a silicon "stamp" that presses on to a polystyrene-based polymer film, producing nanopillars that are extremely long and thin, about 3 microns in height. The leading company in this technology is Hitachi's Advanced Research Laboratory. Researchers and ventures in the US and Europe are pushing ahead with their own nanostamping technologies, including Molecular Imprints Inc (Austin, Texas) and Nanonex Inc (Monmouth Junction, NJ).

The only other technology that comes close to Hitachi's in terms of size is Princeton University's laser-assisted direct imprint technique, which can produce imprinted holes down to 6 nm. The Nanometer Consortium at Lund University in Sweden has developed techniques to direct self-assembly of nanowhiskers. This nano-imprint lithography

(NIL) technique can make stamps with features of less than 20 nm in diameter, and perhaps close to 1:100 in aspect ratio or even larger when optimized. Lund is partnering with Obducat AB in Sweden, to sell NIL machines commercially. Potential applications are in drug discovery and diagnostics.

Nanopores

Nanopores are tiny structures that occur in the cell in nature for specific functions. At the molecular level, specific shapes are created that enable specific chemical tasks to be completed. For examples, some toxic proteins such as alpha hemolysin can embed themselves into cell membranes and induce lethal permeability changes there due to its central pore. This protein consists of seven subunits that join together to form a tunnel through the cell membrane with a well defined pore that narrows from 26 to about 15 – just larger than a single-stranded DNA molecule (van de Goor 2004). The first proposed application was DNA sequencing by measuring the size of nanopore, application of an electric potential across the membrane and waiting for DNA to migrate through the pore to enable one to measure the difference between bases in the sequence. This is tricky as the pore is very small with a diameter of less 1/100th of the wavelength of visible light.

Protein engineering has applied to ion channels and pores and protein as well as non-protein nanopores have been constructed (Bayley and Jayasinghe 2004). Engineered nanopores have potential applications in molecular diagnostics. Agilent Laboratories (Palo Alto, CA) is collaborating with Harvard University (Cambridge, MA) to develop nanopore technology for analysis of nucleic acids that converts strings of nucleotides directly into electronic signatures. A membrane with nanometer diameter channels called nanopores separate two solutions. When a current is applied across the membrane, charged biomolecules migrate through the pores. As each nucleotide passes through the nanopore, an electric signature is produced that characterizes it because the size of the nanopore allows only a single nucleic acid strand to pass through it at one time. Concept of nanopore-based sequencing is shown in Figure 2-2.

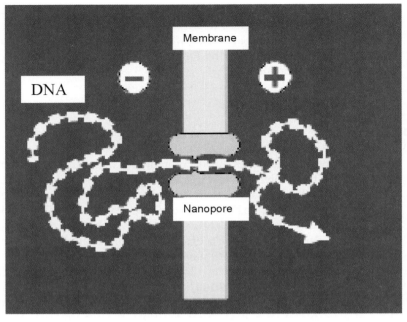

Figure 2-2: Concept of nanopore-based sequencing

When a current is applied across the membrane, charged biomolecules migrate through the pores. As each nucleotide passes through the nanopore, an electric signature is produced that characterizes it because the size of the nanopore allows only a single nucleic acid strand to pass through it at one time.

Bacterial magnetic particles

Magnetic bacteria synthesize intracellular magnetosomes that impart a cellular swimming behavior referred to as magnetotaxis. The magnetic structures, magnetosomes, aligned in chains are postulated to function as biological compass needles allowing the bacterium to migrate along redox gradients through the Earth's geomagnetic field lines. Despite the discovery of this unique group of microorganisms several years ago, the mechanisms of magnetic crystal biomineralization have yet to be fully elucidated. A lipid bilayer membrane of approximately 2-4 nm in thickness encapsulates individual magnetosomes (50-100 nm in diameter). Magnetosomes are also referred to as bacterial magnetic particles (BMPs) to distinguish them from artificial magnetic particles (AMPs). The aggregation of BMPs can be easily dispersed in aqueous solutions compared with AMPs because of the enclosing organic membrane.

BMPs have potential applications in the interdisciplinary fields of nanobiotechnology, medicine and environmental management

(Matsunaga and Okamura 2003). The use of BMPs in immunoassays enables the separation of bound and free analytes by applying a magnetic field. Proteins can be attached covalently to solid supports such as BMPs that prevents desorption of the antibodies during an assay. Large scale production of functionally active antibodies or enzymes expressed on BMP membranes can be accomplished.

Protein-nanoparticle combination

Proteins come in many handy shapes and sizes, which make them major players in biological systems. Chaperonins are ring-shaped proteins found in all living organisms where they play an essential role in stabilizing proteins and facilitating protein folding. A chaperon can be adapted in bacterial protein for technological applications by coaxing it to combine with individual luminescent semiconductor nanoparticles (Ishii et al 2003). In bacteria, this chaperonin protein takes in and re-folds denatured proteins in order to return them to their original useful shapes. Cadmium sulfite nanoparticles emit light as long as they are isolated from each other; encasing the nanoparticles in the protein keeps the tiny particles apart. The biological fuel molecule ATP releases the nanoparticles from the protein tubes, freeing the particles to clump together, which quenches the light.

The protein-nanoparticle combination could be used to detect ATP, according to the researchers. The researchers are working on using the combination to detect specific ATP concentrations. They are also working on coaxing the protein to capture and release organic molecules. This blend of nanotechnology and molecular biology could lead to new bioresponsive electronic nanodevices and biosensors very different from the artificial molecular systems currently available. This ability would make the proteins good candidates for drug carriers. The protein-nanoparticle combination could be used in practical applications in three to five years.

Production techniques for nanoparticles

A large variety of techniques are used for production of nanoparticles. The oldest method is milling or grinding and this process has produced nanoparticles for a long time before the nano dimension of the particles was even recognized. Most of the methods for production of nanoparticles fall into three categories: milling, vapor condensation and chemical synthesis.

Vapor condensation. Vaporization followed by condensation is used for making metallic and ceramic nanoparticles. Inert gases are used to prevent oxidation. Variation of this method includes vapor deposition. This technique allows a better control over particle size and reduces contamination.

Chemical synthesis. This is the most widely used method and involves growing nanoparticles in a liquid medium. It is used for making quantum dots whose mechanical properties rather than size is responsible for unique properties although the two are linked.

Milling or grinding. This is still used for materials where vaporization or chemical synthesis techniques cannot be applied. The properties of resulting nanoparticles depend on the milling material, milling time and atmospheric conditions.

Several new techniques are evolving for manufacture of nanoparticles. These include the following:

- Use of supercritical fluids with properties that are between those of fluids and gases as media for metal particle growth

- Electrodeposit process

- Use of microwave and ultrasound

- Biomimetics or mimicking biology, e.g., yeast cells make cadmium sulfide nanoparticles.

Coating and chemical modifications are areas for innovations in nanoparticle manufacture. For example, Ferrofluids involve magnetite particles that are approximately 10 nm in diameter and are coated with graphite as a stabilizer material. Important considerations in the manufacture of nanoparticles for biotechnology applications are:

- Capacity for production in high volume for applications such as in pharmaceutical industry

- Control over particle size

- Prevention of contamination

Nanomaterials for biolabeling

Nanomaterials are suitable for biolabeling. Nanoparticles usually form the core in nanobiomaterials. However, in order to interact with biological target, a biological or molecular coating or layer acting as an interface needs to be attached to the nanoparticle. Coatings that make the nanoparticles biocompatible include antibodies, biopolymers or monolayers of small molecules. A nanobiomaterial may be in the form of nanovesicle surrounded by a membrane or a layer. The shape is more often spherical but cylindrical, plate-like and other shapes are possible. The size and size distribution might be important in some cases, for example if penetration through a pore structure of a cellular membrane is required. The size is critical when quantum-sized effects are used to control material properties. A tight control of the average particle size and a narrow distribution of sizes allow creating very efficient fluorescent probes that emit narrow light in a very wide range of wavelengths. This helps with creating biomarkers with many and well distinguished colors. The core itself might have several layers and be multifunctional. For example, combining magnetic and luminescent layers one can both detect and manipulate the particles.

The core particle is often protected by several monolayers of inert material, for example silica. Organic molecules that are adsorbed or chemisorbed on the surface of the particle are also used for this purpose. The same layer might act as a biocompatible material. However, more often an additional layer of linker molecules is required that has reactive groups at both ends. One group is aimed at attaching the linker to the nanoparticle surface and the other is used to bind various biocompatible substances such as antibodies depending on the function required by the application.

Efforts to improve the performance of immunoassays and immunosensors by incorporating different kinds of nanostructures have gained considerable momentum over the last decade. Most of the studies focus on artificial, particulate marker systems, both organic and inorganic. Inorganic nanoparticle labels based on noble metals, semiconductor quantum dots and nanoshells appear to be the most versatile systems for these bioanalytical applications of nanophotonics. The underlying detection procedures are more commonly based on optical techniques. These include nanoparticle applications generating signals as diverse as static and time-resolved luminescence, one- and two-photon absorption, Raman and Rayleigh scattering as well as surface plasmon resonance and others. In general, all efforts are aimed to achieve one or more of the following goals (Seydack 2005):

- Lowering of detection limits (if possible, down to single-molecule level)

- Parallel integration of multiple signals (multiplexing)

- Signal amplification by several orders of magnitude

- Prevention of photobleaching effects with concomitant maintenance of antigen binding specificity and sensitivity.

Potential benefits of using nanoparticles and nanodevices include an expanded range of label multiplexing (Fortina et al 2005). Various nanomaterials for biolabeling are shown in Table 2-4. Some examples are described briefly in the following text and other parts of the book.

Table 2-4: Nanomaterials for biolabeling

Label/reporter	Characteristics	Function/ applications
Electrogenerated chemiluminescence	Tris(2,2´-bipyridyl)ruthenium(II) molecular labels	Nanoscale bioassay
Europium nanoparticles	Biolabeling by highly sensitive time-resolved fluorescence bioassays	Nanoparticle-labeled streptavidin for sandwich-type time-resolved fluoroimmunoassays of CEA and HBsAg in human sera (Tan et al 2004).
Europium(III)-chelate-doped nanoparticles	Combined with selection of high affinity monoclonal antibodies coated on label particles and microtitration wells.	The sensitivity for virus particle detection was improved by three orders of magnitude compared to immunofluorometric assays (Valanne et al 2005).
Fluorescent color-changing dyes	3-hydroxychromone derivatives that exhibit two fluorescence bands as a result of excited-state intramolecular proton transfer reaction	Biosensors
Lanthanide chelates	Fluorescence probes or labels based on the microsecond time-resolved fluorescence measurement techniques	Highly sensitive detections of various biological molecules.
Luminescent core/shell nanohybride	Luminescent rare earth ions in a nanosized Gd_2O_3 core (3.5 nm) and FITC molecules entrapped within in a polysiloxane shell (2.5-10 nm).	Two different luminescence emissions: (1) FITC under standard illumination; (2) Tb^{3+} under high-energy source giving highly photostable luminescence
Nanogold® labels (Nanoprobe Inc)	Unlike nanogold particles, gold labels are uncharged molecules, which are cross-linked to specific sites on biomolecules	Nanogold® labels have a range and versatility, which is not available with colloidal nanogold particles
Plasmon resonant nanoparticles	Scatter light with tremendous efficiency	Ultrabright nanosized labels for biological applications, replacing other labeling methods such as fluorescence.
Multicolor quantum-dot (QD)end-labeling	Multicolor fluorescence microscopy using conjugated QDs	Detection of single DNA molecules

SERS (Surface-enhanced Raman Scattering)-based nanotags (Nanoplex Technologies)	A metal nanoparticle where each type of tag exploits the Raman spectrum of a different small molecule and SERS bands are 1/50th the width of fluorescent bands.	Allow for greater multiplexed analyte quantification than current fluorescence-based quantitation tags.

Quantum dots as labels

The unique optical properties of QDs make them appealing as in vivo and in vitro fluorophores in a variety of biological investigations, in which traditional fluorescent labels based on organic molecules fall short of providing long-term stability and simultaneous detection of multiple signals (Medintz et al 2005). The ability to make QDs water soluble and target them to specific biomolecules has led to promising applications in cellular labeling, deep-tissue imaging, assay labeling and as efficient fluorescence resonance energy transfer donors.

A new method for the detection of surface-attached DNA molecules by fluorescence microscopy has been described (Crut et al 2005). Biotin- and/or digoxigenin-modified DNA fragments are covalently linked at both extremities of a DNA molecule via sequence-specific hybridization and ligation. After the modified DNA molecules have been stretched on a glass surface, their ends are visualized by multicolor fluorescence microscopy using conjugated quantum dots (QD). The position and orientation of individual DNA molecules can be inferred with good efficiency from the QD fluorescence signals alone. This is achieved by selecting QD pairs that have the distance and direction expected for the combed DNA molecules. Direct observation of single DNA molecules in the absence of DNA staining agent opens new possibilities in the fundamental study of DNA–protein interactions. This approach can be applied for the use of QD for nucleic acid detection and analysis.

Nanogold labels

Unlike conventional immunogold probes, in which colloidal gold particles are electrostatically adsorbed to antibodies and proteins, Nanoprobe Inc's gold labels are uncharged molecules which are cross-linked to specific sites on biomolecules. This gives the probes a range and versatility which is not available with colloidal gold. These labels can be attached to any molecule with a reactive group – proteins, peptides, oligonucleotides, small molecules and lipids – for detection and localization. Other labels can be combined with gold labels;

FluoroNanogold probes combine Nanogold® and fluorescein into a single probe for imaging a specimen both by fluorescence and electron microscopy. New probes can be engineered based on any fragment of a naturally occurring biomolecule, and the label can be positioned away from the binding site so it does not interfere with binding.

Silver nanoparticle labels

A novel, sensitive electrochemical DNA hybridization detection assay uses silver nanoparticles as oligonucleotide labeling tags (Cao et al 2002). The assay relies on the hybridization of the target DNA with the silver nanoparticle-oligonucleotide DNA probe, followed by the release of the silver metal atoms anchored on the hybrids by oxidative metal dissolution and the indirect determination of the solubilized Ag^I ions by anodic stripping voltammetry. The experimental variables, including the surface coverage of the target oligonucleotide, the duration of the silver dissolution steps and the parameters of the electrochemical stripping measurement of the Ag^I ions, were optimized. High sensitivity of the stripping metal analysis at the microelectrode, combined with the large number of Ag^I ions released from each DNA hybrid, enables detection at levels as low as 0.5 pmol L^{-1} of the target oligonucleotides.

Silica nanoparticles for labeling antibodies

Luminescent silicon dioxide nanoparticles with size of 50 nm containing rhodamine (R-SiO2) have been synthesized by sol-gel method. These particles can emit intense and stable room temperature phosphorescence signals. An immune reaction between goat-anti-human IgG antibody labeled with R-SiO2 and human IgG has been demonstrated on polyamide membrane quantitatively, and the phosphorescence intensity was enhanced after the immunoreactions (Jia-Ming et al 2005). This is the basis of a room temperature phosphorescence immunoassay for the determination of human IgG using an antibody labeled with the nanoparticles containing binary luminescent molecules. This method is sensitive, accurate and precise.

Lissamine rhodamine B sulfonylchloride and other dyes can be covalently bound to and contained in spherical silica nanoparticles (30–80 nm). Compared to organic molecular markers these fluorophore hybrid silica particles exhibit superior photostability and detection sensitivity. An immunoassay method for detecting a trace level (down to 0.1 ng/mL) of hepatitis B surface antigen was successfully developed on this basis (Yang et al 2004).

Organic nanoparticles as biolabels

The use of organic nonpolymeric nanoparticles as biolabels was not considered to be promising or have any advantage over established metallic or polymeric probes. Problems include quenching of fluorescence in organic dye crystals, colloidal stability and solubility in aqueous environments but some of these can be circumvented. Labels have been constructed by milling and suspending a fluorogenic hydrophobic precursor, fluorescein diacetate (FDA), in sodium dodecyl sulfate (SDS). Thus, a negative surface charge is introduced, rendering the particles (500 nm) colloidally stable and minimizing leakage of FDA molecules into surrounding water. Now it has been shown that the polyelectrolyte multilayer architechture is not vital for the operability of this assay format. Instead of SDS and multilayers the adsorption of only one layer of an amphiphilic polymeric detergent, e.g. an alkylated poly(ethylene imine), is sufficient to stabilize the system and to provide an interface for the antibody attachment (Bruemmel et al 2004). This is the basis of a technology marketed under the name "ImmunoSuperNova®" by 8sens.biognostic AG, Germany. In this the reaction of the analyte molecule with the capture antibody is followed by an incubation step with the antibody-nanoparticle (IgG-FDA) conjugate, which serves as detector. After some washing steps an organic release solvent is added, dissolving the particle and converting FDA into fluorescein.

Applications of nanotechnology in life sciences

Life sciences are the testing ground for many new biotechnologies. Nanobiotechnology is a good example. Much of the research in life sciences is directly relevant to diagnostic applications described in the following chapters.

Investigative methods of nanotechnology have made inroads into uncovering fundamental biological processes, including self-assembly, cellular processes, and systems biology (such as neural systems). Key advances have been made in the ability to make measurements at the sub-cellular level and in understanding the cell as a highly organized, self-repairing, self-replicating, information-rich molecular machine. Single-molecule measurements are shedding light on the dynamics and mechanistic properties of molecular biomachines, both in vivo and in vitro, allowing the direct investigation of molecular motors, enzyme reactions, protein dynamics, DNA transcription and cell signaling. It has also been possible to measure the chemical composition within a single cell in vivo. Micro total analysis systems, using molecular manipulation on nanoscale, offer the potential for highly efficient, simultaneous analysis of a large number of biologically important molecules in genomic, proteomic and metabolic studies.

The physical sciences offer tools for synthesis and fabrication of devices for measuring the characteristics of cells and sub-cellular components, and of materials useful in cell and molecular biology; biology offers a window into the most sophisticated collection of functional nanostructures that exists. Particles made of semiconductors at the nanoscale are already used in the electronic and information technology industries. For example, the active part of a single transistor on a Pentium silicon chip is a few tenths of a nanometer in size. The semiconductor laser used to read digital information on a CD or DVD has an active layer of similar dimensions. Creating the ability to import such electronic functions into the cell and meshing them with biological functions could open tremendous new possibilities, both for basic biological sciences and for medical and therapeutic applications. For example quantum dots (QDs) are used by life science researchers as tiny beacons or markers, allowing them to easily see individual genes, nucleic acids, proteins or small molecules.

Nanobiotechnology and systems biology

Systems biology which is defined as the biology of dynamic interacting networks (Weston and Hood 2004). It is also referred to as pathway, network, or integrative biology. An analysis of the structure and dynamics of network of interacting elements provides insights that are not obvious from analysis of the isolated components of the system. Proteomics plays an important role in systems biology because most biological systems involve proteins. Systems biology is providing new challenges for advancing science and technology. Analyses of pathways may provide new insight into the understanding of disease processes, developing more efficient biomarkers and understanding mechanisms of action of drugs. Nanobiotechnology will play an important role in the study of systems biology by:

- Providing refined tools for the study of proteomics

- Nanotechnology provides real-time single particle tracing in living cells.

- Nanotechnology will facilitate dissecting of signaling pathways.

Nanobiology and the cell

It is perhaps superfluous to use the term 'nanobiology' because cell is the smallest unit alive. Molecules in the cell are organized in nanometer scale dimensions. Visualizing the dynamic change in these molecules and studying the function of cells is one of the challenges in nanobiology. A single molecule is the ultimate nanostructure. Single molecule microscopy and spectroscopy are some of the techniques used to study single molecules.

The objective is to gain a detailed knowledge about biochemical processes occurring locally in the cell nucleus, which is a prerequisite for a comprehensive understanding of genome function. The combination of a resolution range of a few nanometers, high penetrating power, analytical sensitivity, and compatibility with wet specimens allows x-ray microscopy and scanning x-ray microscopy of whole cells. The spatial resolution of 20 nm reached up to now is much better than that of current conventional light microscopes. To further our understanding of chromosome biology and nuclear function, it is essential to develop techniques that enable the measurement of structures inside the living cell with a spatial resolution down to the scale of 10 nm. The ability to work with an individual cell using nanotechnology is very promising as the single cell is an ideal sensor for detecting various chemical and biochemical processes.

Live cell imaging and a novel fluorescence assay have been used to visualize the formation of clathrin–coated vesicles at single clathrin–coated pits (CCP) with a time resolution of seconds (Merrifield et al 2005). This revealed how proteins linked to the actin, a part of the molecular motor, are transported to sites of coated pit. Disturbing actin polymerization with the toxin latrunculin B, a toxin found in Red Sea sponge, drastically reduces the efficiency of membrane scission and affects many aspects of CCP dynamics. The novel assay used in this study can be applied for drug screening. It has been shown that particles in the size range of tens to hundreds of nanometers can enter or exit cells via wrapping even in the absence of clathrin or caveolin coats, and an optimal particles size exists for the smallest wrapping time (Gao et al 2005).

Study of complex biological systems

Nanotechnology holds great promise for the analysis of complex processes inside living cells. It is anticipated to provide new tools to study the responses of different naturally occurring and genetically altered cell types and extend the approaches for monitoring cell behavior and activity in embryos, differentiated tissues, and organs as well as physiological systems. In addition to biological sensors that will be able to measure single molecule behavior, nanodevices are presently being developed that can be used to relocate various components inside the cell nucleus. This will allow different regions in the nucleus to be probed and manipulated to study various processes, such as their permissiveness for transcription. This will likely open direct approaches for investigating structure-function relationships by perturbing the local organization of the genome and determining its effect on function. A most promising method for nanomanipulation in living cells is the use of magnetic nanoparticles that are microinjected into the nucleus of living cells. Such particles can be functionalized by the covalent attachment of selected molecules, e.g., specific proteins. Recently developed magnetic tweezers, in combination with high-resolution microscopy, would allow one to move such nanoparticles at will inside living cells, thereby changing local genome structure. Nanoprobes in the nucleus could be used to monitor changes in chromosome arrangement associated with changes in gene expression.

Biosensing of cellular responses

Cells represent the minimum functional and integrating communicable unit of living systems. Cultured cells both transduce and transmit a variety of chemical and physical signals, i.e., production of specific substances and proteins, throughout their life cycle within specific tissues and organs. Such cellular responses might be usefully employed as parameters to obtain chemical information for both pharmaceutical and chemical safety, and drug efficacy profiles in vitro as a screening tool. However, such cellular signals are very weak and not easily detected with conventional analytical methods. By using micro- and nanobiotechnology methods integrated on a biochip, a higher sensitivity and signal amplification has been developed for cellular biosensing (Haruyama 2003). Nanotechnology is rapidly evolving to open new combinations of methods with improved technical performance, helping to resolve challenging bioanalytical problems including sensitivity, signal resolution and specificity by interfacing these technologies in small volumes in order to confirm specific cellular signals. Integration of cell signals in both rapid time and small space, and importantly, between different cell populations (communication and systems modeling) will permit many more valuable measurements of the dynamic aspects of cell responses to various chosen stimuli and their feedback. This represents the future for cell-based biosensing.

Genetically encoded nanosensors have been developed to monitor glutamate levels inside and at the surface of living cells using the fluorescent indicator protein for glutamate (FLIPE), which consists of the glutamate/aspartate binding protein ybeJ from *Escherichia coli* fused to two variants of the green fluorescent protein (Okumoto et al 2005). The sensors respond to extracellular glutamate with a reversible concentration-dependent decrease in FRET efficiency. FLIPE nanosensors can be used for real-time monitoring of glutamate metabolism in living cells, in tissues, or in intact organisms, providing tools for studying metabolism or for drug discovery.

3. NANOMOLECULAR DIAGNOSTICS

Abstract

This is the main chapter describing the use of nanobiotechnologies as applied to molecular diagnostics under the term "nanodiagnostics". Classification of these technologies includes a variety of approaches starting with those that improve the conventional molecular diagnostics such as polymerase chain reaction (PCR). Some technologies are based on nanoparticles whereas others use nanosensors and nanotechnologies on biochips. Most commonly used nanoparticles are quantum dots and gold nanoparticles. Magnetic nanoparticles have been used for imaging in vivo along with magnetic resonance imaging (MRI). Nanobarcodes, with various submicrometer striping patterns, may be readily distinguished in an optical microscope and are useful for bioanalytical measurements.

Introduction

Nanomolecular diagnostics is the use of nanobiotechnology in molecular diagnostics and can be termed "nanodiagnostics" (Jain 2003a). Numerous nanodevices and nanosystems for sequencing single molecules of DNA are feasible. It seems quite likely that there will be numerous applications of inorganic nanostructures in biology and medicine as markers. Given the inherent nanoscale of receptors, pores, and other functional components of living cells, the detailed monitoring and analysis of these components will be made possible by the development of a new class of nanoscale probes. Biological tests measuring the presence or activity of selected substances become quicker, more sensitive and more flexible when certain nanoscale particles are put to work as tags or labels. Nanotechnology will improve the sensitivity and integration of analytical methods to yield a more coherent evaluation of life processes.

The chemical modification and global amplification of the nucleic acid samples are achieved by PCR (see Chapter 1), which can introduce artifacts caused by the preferential amplification of certain sequences. Alternative label-free methods include surface plasmon resonance and quartz crystal microbalance, which rely on mass detection. Nanotechnologies also provide label-free detection. Nanotechnology is thus being applied to overcome some of the limitations of biochip technology. This chapter focuses on the applications of nanotechnologies for molecular diagnostics.

Classification of nanotechnologies used for molecular diagnostics

It is difficult to classify such a variety of technologies but various nanotechnologies with potential applications in molecular diagnostics are listed in Table 3-1. Nanotechnology on a chip was described in Chapter 2. Some of the other technologies will be described briefly in the following text using examples of commercial products.

Table 3-1: Nanotechnologies with potential applications in molecular diagnostics

Nanotechnology to improve polymerase chain reaction (PCR)
Nano-JETA™ real-time PCR
Nanotechnology on a chip
Microfluidic chips for nanoliter volumes: NanoChip
Optical readout of nanoparticle labels
NanoArrays
Protein nanoarrays
Nanoparticle technologies
Gold particles
Nanobarcodes
Magnetic nanoparticles: Ferrofluids, supramagnetic particles combined with MRI
Quantum dot technology
Nanoparticle probes
Nanowires
Nanopore technology
Measuring length of DNA fragments in a high-throughput manner
DNA fingerprinting
Haplotyping
Cantilever arrays
Multiple combined tests (such as protein and DNA) to be performed on the same disposable chip
Prostate specific antigen binding to antibody
DNA nanomachines for molecular diagnostics
Nanoparticle-based immunoassays
DNA-protein and nanoparticle conjugates
Resonance Light Scattering technology
Nanosensors
Living spores as nanodetectors
Nanopore nanosensors
Quartz nanobalance DNA sensor

PEBBLE (Probes Encapsulated by Biologically Localized Embedding) nanosensors
Nanosensor glucose monitor
Photostimulated luminescence in nanoparticles
Optical biosensors: Surface plasmon resonance technology

Rationale of nanotechnology for molecular diagnostics

Numerous nanodevices and nanosystems for sequencing single molecules of DNA are feasible. It is likely that there will be numerous applications of inorganic nanostructures in biology and medicine as markers:

- Nanoscale probes would be suitable for detailed analysis of receptors, pores, and other components of living cells that are on a nanoscale.

- Nanoscale particles, used as tags or labels, increase the sensitivity, speed and flexibility of biological tests measuring the presence or activity of selected substances

- Nanotechnology will improve the sensitivity and integration of analytical methods to yield a more coherent evaluation of life processes.

Nanotechnology to improve polymerase chain reaction

Polymerase chain reaction (PCR) is still the most commonly used technology used in molecular diagnostics. One of its important refinements is real-time PCR. Acrongenomics is developing Nano-JETA™ technology platform to develop the Nano-JETA™ real-time PCR. It was validated in a clinical study to detect Ep-CAM gene and beta-actin (internal control) in peripheral blood of patients suffering from breast and colon cancer with histologically and cytologically verified pathology. Nano-JETA™, using 8 µL of sample and 13 cycles, was compared with conventional real time PCR that used 45 cycles and 25 µL of sample. Results revealed that in the case of beta-actin (internal control) both protocols exhibited 100% specificity. Beta-actin was detectable from the 16th to 18th cycle when using conventional real-time PCR, while only 1 single cycle was required with Nano-JETA(TM) real-time PCR. Regarding sensitivity, conventional real-time PCR detected 10 to the 4th cancer cells, while requiring 22 to 32 cycles. Nano-JETA real-time PCR was found to be hundred times more sensitive than conventional real-time PCR.

Nanotechnology for separation of DNA fragments

A technology using core-shell type nanospheres and nanoparticle medium in conjunction with a pressurization technique was used to carry out separations of a wide range of DNA fragments with high speed and high resolution during microchip electrophoresis (Tabuchi et al 2004). DNA fragments up to 15 kilo base pairs were successfully analyzed within 100 seconds without observing any saturation in migration rates. Optimal pressure conditions and concentrations of packed nanospheres are considered to be important for achieving improved DNA separations.

Nanoparticles for molecular diagnostics

Gold particles

Bits of DNA and Raman-active dyes can be attached to gold particles no larger than 13 nanometers in diameter. The gold nanoparticles assemble onto a sensor surface only in the presence of a complementary target. If a patterned sensor surface of multiple DNA strands is used, the technique can detect millions of different DNA sequences simultaneously. The current non-optimized detection limit of this method is 20 femtomolars. Gold nanoparticles are particularly good labels for sensors because a variety of analytical techniques can be used to detect them, including optical absorption, fluorescence, Raman scattering, atomic and magnetic force, and electrical conductivity. Gold nanoparticles combined with a Raman spectroscopy technique to detect life-threatening bacteria and viruses such as anthrax and HIV. Raman approach could replace PCR and fluorescent tags commonly used today. The detection system also relies on chips dotted with DNA. If the targeted disease exists in the sample, its DNA will bind onto the complementary strands of DNA on the chip and gold particle. The chip is treated with silver-based solution, which coats the nanoparticles. When exposed to a light scanner, the coating enhances the signal enough to detect minute amounts of DNA. Since the Raman band is narrower than the fluorescent band, it allows more dyes to detect more targets quickly. If the sequence of interest is present in the sample, it will bind to the DNA and cause the solution to change color. Labeling oligonucleotide targets with gold nanoparticle rather than fluorophore probes substantially alters the melting profiles of the targets from an array substrate. A nanoparticle-based DNA detection system is 10 times more sensitive and 100,000 times more specific than current genomic detection systems (Park et al 2002).

DNA can be coaxed to aggregate and separate gold nanoparticles on demand (Hazarika et al 2004). The method uses two single-strand sequences of DNA each of which is attached to a gold nanoparticle, and a third single strand that has three sections. The first two sections of the third strand match up with each of the nanoparticle strands, gluing them together so that the gold nanoparticles they carry are positioned close together. The nanoparticles can be pulled apart again using a third type of DNA strand that matches up with the entire glue strand of DNA. This glue removal strand first attaches to the free third section of the glue strand, then continues until the entire glue strand is pulled free. The method could be used in sensors that detect biological substances. It could also be used in programmable materials whose properties can be changed by the addition of a piece of DNA.

Quantum dots for molecular diagnostics

There is considerable interest in the use of quantum dots (QDs) as inorganic fluorophores, owing to the fact that they offer significant advantages over conventionally used fluorescent markers. For example, QDs have fairly broad excitation spectra – from ultraviolet to red – that can be tuned depending on their size and composition. At the same time, QDs have narrow emission spectra, making it possible to resolve the emissions of different nanoparticles simultaneously and with minimal overlap. Finally, QDs are highly resistant to degradation, and their fluorescence is remarkably stable. Advantages of QD technology are:

- Simple excitation. Lasers are not required.

- Simple instrumentation

- Availability of red/infrared colors enables whole blood assays

- High sensitivity

QDs have been used as possible alternatives to the dyes for tagging viruses and cancer cells. A major challenge is that QDs have an oily surface, whereas the cellular environment is water-based. Attempts are being made to modify the surface chemistry of QDs so that they interact with water-friendly molecules like proteins and DNA. The current goal is to develop QDs that can target a disease site and light it up. This can someday lead to an integrated system that will also use the QDs to diagnose as well to deliver drug therapies to the disease site. QDs can be designed to emit light at any wavelength from the infrared to visible to ultraviolet. This enables the use of a large number of colors and thus multiplexed assays can be performed. Potential applications of QDs in molecular diagnostics can be summarized as follows:

- Cancer

- Genotyping

- Whole blood assays

- Multiplexed diagnostics

- DNA mapping

- Immunoassays and antibody tagging

- Detection of pathogenic microorganisms

Quantum dots for detection of pathogenic microorganisms

QDs have been used as fluorescent labels in immunoassays for quantitative detection of foodborne pathogenic bacteria (Yang and Lee 2005). *Salmonella typhimurium* cells were separated from chicken carcass wash water using anti-Salmonella antibody coated magnetic beads and reacted to secondary biotin-labeled anti-Salmonella antibody. QDs coated with streptavidin were added to react with biotin on the secondary antibody. Measurement of the intensity of fluorescence produced by quantum dots provided a quantitative method for microbial detection.

QDs can be used for ultrasensitive viral detection of a small number of microorganisms. QD-based tests can detect as low as 100 copies of hepatitis and HIV viral RNA. Applications of tests based on QDs for clinical diagnosis of viral infections are described in Chapter 6.

Quantum dots for detection of cell surface proteins

Antibody-based labeling has been used for targeting quantum dots (QDs) to cells but there are two problems: the size of the QD conjugate after antibody attachment and the instability of many antibody-antigen interactions. One way to overcome these limitations is to tag the mammalian cell surface proteins with acceptor peptide (AP), which can be biotinylated by biotin ligase added to the medium, while endogenous proteins remain unmodified (Howarth et al 2005). The biotin group then serves as a handle for targeting streptavidin-conjugated-QDs. QDs have been targeted to cell surface cyan fluorescent protein and epidermal growth factor receptor in HeLa cells and to alpha-amino-3-hydroxy-5-methyl-4-isoxazolepropionate (AMPA) receptors in neurons. Labeling is specific for the AP-tagged protein, and is highly sensitive. Thus biotin ligase labeling provides a specific, rapid, and generally applicable method for detecting and tracking cell surface proteins.

Disguising quantum dots as proteins for cell entry as probes

A unique new coating for inorganic particles at the nanoscale can disguise quantum dots (QDs) as proteins - a process that allows particles to function as probes to penetrate the cell and light up individual proteins inside, creating the potential for application in a wide range of drug development and diagnostic tool applications (Michalet et al 2005).

The organic coatings - short chains of peptides - can be used to disguise QDs, quantum rods and quantum wires so effectively that the cells mistake them for proteins, even when the coatings are used on particles that are inorganic and possibly even toxic. The new coatings enables the solubilization and introduction into the cell of different color QDs that can all be excited by a single blue light source. In addition to the capacity to paint and observe many different proteins with separate colors, QDs can be used for the ultimate detection sensitivity: observing a single molecule. Until now, tracking and following a single protein molecule in the cell has been extremely difficult.

This method, along with a fluorescence microscope and high-sensitivity imaging cameras, enables the tracking a single protein tagged with a fluorescent QD inside a living cell in three dimensions and within a few nanometers of accuracy. Particles disguised with the peptide coatings can enter a cell without affecting its basic functioning. Since the peptide-coated QDs are small, they have easy and rapid entry through the cell membrane. In addition, since multiple peptides of various lengths and functions could be deposited on the same single QD, it would be feasible to create smart probes with multiple functions. It might enable the creation of a hybrid nanoparticle that could be specifically targeted to identify and destroy cancer cells in the body.

Imaging of living tissue with quantum dots

Tiny blood vessels, viewed beneath a mouse's skin with a newly developed application of multi-photon microscopy, appear so bright and vivid in high-resolution images that researchers can see the vessel walls ripple with each heartbeat. Cornell Researchers, in collaboration with Quantum Dot Corporation have shown that capillaries many hundreds of microns below the skin of living mice were illuminated in unprecedented detail using fluorescence imaging labels, quantum dots, circulating through the bloodstream (Larson et al 2003). This is a new approach to using quantum dots for biological studies of living animals. Although there are easier ways to take a mouse's pulse, this level of resolution and high signal-to-noise illustrates how useful multi-photon microscopy with quantum dots can become in biological research for tracking cells and visualizing tissue structures deep inside living animals. Monitoring of vascular changes in malignant tumors is a possible application. This research will pave the way for many new non-invasive in-vivo imaging methods using quantum dots.

Carbohydrate-encapsulated QD can be used for medical imaging. Certain carbohydrates, especially those included on tumor glycoproteins are known to have affinity for certain cell types and this can be exploited for medical imaging. Conjugating luminescent QDs with target specific glycans permits efficient imaging of the tissue to which the glycans bind with high affinity. Accurate imaging of primary and metastatic tumors is of primary importance in disease management. Second generation QDs contain the glycan ligands and PEG of varying chain lengths. The PEG modifications produce QDs that maintain high luminescence while reducing non-specific cell binding.

Procedures have been developed for using QDs to label live cells and to demonstrate their use for long-term multicolor imaging (Jaiswal et al 2003). The two approaches are endocytic uptake of QDs and selective labeling of cell surface proteins with QDs conjugated to antibodies. These approaches should permit the simultaneous study of multiple cells over long periods of time as they proceed through growth and development. Use of avidin permits stable conjugation of the QDs to ligands, antibodies or other molecules that can be biotinylated, whereas the use of proteins fused to a positively charged peptide or oligohistidine peptide obviates the need for biotinylating the target molecule. A procedure has been described for the bioconjugation of QDs and specific labeling of both intracellular and cell-surface proteins (Jaiswal et al 2004). For generalized cellular labeling, QDs not conjugated to a specific biomolecule may be used.

Quantum dots for cancer diagnosis

In a novel probe, QDs are bound to gold nanoparticles (AuNPs) via a proteolytically degradable peptide sequence to suppress luminescence and signal amplification occurs upon interaction with a targeted proteolytic enzyme (Chang et al 2005). A 71% reduction in luminescence was achieved with conjugation of AuNPs to QDs. Release of AuNPs by peptide cleavage restored radiative QD photoluminescence. These probes can be customized for targeted degradation simply by changing the sequence of the peptide linker and may be useful for imaging in cancer diagnosis.

By attaching a QD to a molecule that will target a specific type of cancer, QDs can accumulate in the tumor, which will light up. Another limitation is that light penetration into the body is limited; one can screen for superficial cancers but it is difficult to reach cancers located deep in the body. For example, screening for skin, breast or prostate cancer might be possible but the technology might not work for lung or colon cancer.

Using quantum dots that emit near-infrared light, researchers have developed an improved method for performing sentinel lymph node biopsy, which depends on illuminating lymph nodes during cancer surgery (Kim et al 2004). The infrared quantum dots were developed and synthesized at the MIT department of chemistry in collaboration with Quantum Dot Corporation. The first challenge was that the particles had to be rendered soluble, which was achieved by using a polydentate phosphene coating. The quantum dots were engineered to emit near-infrared light, a part of the spectrum that is transmitted through biological tissue with minimal scattering. The study describes how the quantum dots were injected into live pigs and followed visually to the lymph system just beneath the skin of the animals. The new imaging technique allowed the surgeons to clearly see the target lymph nodes without cutting the animals' skin. Sentinel Lymph Node (SLN) mapping, the surgical technique employed in the study, is a common procedure used to identify the presence of cancer in a single, "sentinel" lymph node, thus avoiding the removal of a patient's entire lymph system. SLN mapping relies on a combination of radioactivity and organic dyes but the technique is inexact during surgery, often leading to removal of much more of the lymph system than necessary, causing unwanted trauma. This study is a significant improvement over the dye/radioactivity method currently used to perform SLN mapping.

Throughout the procedure, the quantum dots were clearly visible using the imaging system, allowing the surgeon to see not only the lymph nodes, but also the underlying anatomy. The imaging system and quantum dots allowed the pathologist to focus on specific parts of the SLN that would be most likely to contain malignant cells, if cancer were present. The imaging system and quantum dots minimized inaccuracies and permitted real-time confirmation of the total removal of the target lymph nodes, drastically reducing the potential for repeated procedures.

SLN mapping has already revolutionized cancer surgery. Near-infrared quantum dots have the potential to improve this important technique even further. Because the dots in the study are composed of heavy metals, which can be toxic, they have not yet been approved for use in humans. The next step is to develop quantum dots that can be used safely in human trials.

Magnetic nanoparticles

Magnetic nanoparticles are a powerful and versatile diagnostic tool in biology and medicine. It is possible to incorporate sufficient amounts of superparamagnetic iron oxide (SPIO) nanoparticles into cells, enabling their detection in vivo using MRI (Bulte et al 2004). Because of their small size, they are easily incorporated into various cell types (stem cells, phagocytes etc) allowing the cells to be tracked in vivo, for example to determine whether stem cells move to the correct target area of the body.

Bound to a suitable antibody, magnetic nanoparticles are used to label specific molecules, structures, or microorganisms. Magnetic immunoassay techniques have been developed in which the magnetic field generated by the magnetically labeled targets is detected directly with a sensitive magnetometer. Binding of antibody to target molecules or disease-causing organism is the basis of several tests. Antibodies labeled with magnetic nanoparticles give magnetic signals on exposure to a magnetic field. Antibodies bound to targets can thus be identified as unbound antibodies disperse in all directions and produce no net magnetic signal.

A novel nanosensor based on magnetic nanoparticles has been developed for rapid screens of telomerase activity in biological samples (Grimm et al 2004). The technique utilizes nanoparticles that, on annealing with telomerase synthesized TTAGGG repeats, switch their magnet state, a phenomenon readily detectable by magnetic readers. High-throughput adaptation of the technique by magnetic resonance imaging allowed processing of hundreds of samples within tens of minutes at ultrahigh sensitivities. Together, these studies establish and validate a novel and powerful tool for rapidly sensing telomerase activity and provide the rationale for developing analogous magnetic nanoparticles for in vivo sensing. Since elevated telomerase levels are found in many malignancies, this technique offers provides access to an attractive target for therapeutic intervention and diagnostic or prognostic purposes.

Ferrofluids

CellTracks™ Technology (Immunicon) is based on patented magnetic nanoparticles called ferrofluids. Ferrofluid consists of a magnetic core surrounded by a polymeric layer coated with antibodies for capturing cells. Ferrofluid particles are colloidal and when mixed with a sample containing the target cells, the antibodies conjugated to the magnetic core bind the antigen associated with the target cells. It is combined with proprietary technologies for cell separation, labeling and analysis. This is in development to screen, diagnose, stage, and monitor cancer based on circulating cancer cells in the blood. Potential applications include isolation of endothelial cells, which may be useful in the management of cancer and cardiovascular disease, and isolation of fungus or bacteria, which may be useful in the management of patients with serious infections.

Super conducting quantum interference device

Superconducting quantum interference device (SQUID), developed at University of California (Berkeley, CA), is a technique for specific, sensitive, quantitative, and rapid detection of biological targets by using super paramagnetic nanoparticles (Quantum Magnetics, San Diego, CA) and a "microscope" based on a high-transition temperature (Chemla et al 2000). In this technique, a mylar film to which the targets have been bound is placed on the microscope alongside SQUID. A suspension of magnetic nanoparticles carrying antibodies directed against the target is added to the mixture in the well, and 1-s pulses of magnetic field are applied parallel to the SQUID. In the presence of this aligning field the nanoparticles develop a net magnetization, which relaxes when the field is turned off. Unbound nanoparticles relax rapidly by Brownian rotation and contribute no measurable signal. Nanoparticles that are bound to the target on the film are immobilized and undergo a slowly decaying magnetic flux, which is detected by the SQUID. The ability to distinguish between bound and unbound labels allows one to run homogeneous assays, which do not require separation and removal of unbound magnetic particles.

Use of nanocrystals in immunohistochemistry

A method has been described for simple convenient preparation of bright, negatively or positively charged, water-soluble CdSe/ZnS core/shell nanocrystals (NCs) and their stabilization in aqueous solution (Sukhanova et al 2004). Single NCs can be detected using a standard epifluorescent microscope, ensuring a detection limit of one molecule coupled with an NC. NC-antibody (Ab) conjugates were tested in dot-blots and exhibited retention of binding capacity within several nanograms of antigen detected. The authors further demonstrated the advantages of NC-Ab conjugates in the immunofluorescent detection and 3D confocal analysis of p-glycoprotein (p-gp), one of the main mediators of the multi-drug resistance phenotype. The labeling of p-gp with NC-Ab conjugates was highly specific. Finally, the authors demonstrated the applicability of NC-Abs conjugates obtained by the method described to specific detection of antigens in paraffin-embedded formaldehyde-fixed cancer tissue specimens, using immunostaining of cytokeratin in skin basal carcinoma as an example. They concluded that the NC-Ab conjugates may serve as easy-to-do, highly sensitive, photostable labels for immunofluorescent analysis, immunohistochemical detection, and 3D confocal studies of membrane proteins and cells.

Bioelectronic assays based on carbon nanotubes

Signal amplification using enzyme multilayers on carbon nanotube (CNT) templates is shown to yield a remarkably sensitive electrochemical detection of proteins and nucleic acids. The electrostatic layer-by-layer (LBL) self-assembly onto CNT carriers maximizes the ratio of enzyme tags per binding event to offer the greatest amplification factor reported so far (Munge et al 2005). Absorption spectroscopy, TEM, and electrochemical characterization confirm the formation of LBL enzyme nanostructures on individual CNT carriers. The enzymatic activity is found to increase with the number of enzyme layers. It can be used for monitoring sandwich hybridization and antibody-antigen interactions in connection with alkaline phosphatase tracers. Amplified bioelectronic assays enable detection of DNA and proteins down to 80 copies and 2000 protein molecules respectively. Given the enormous amplification afforded by the new CNT-LBL biolabel, such route offers great promise for ultrasensitive detection of infectious agents and disease markers.

Study of chromosomes by atomic force microscopy

A better knowledge of biochemical and structural properties of human chromosomes is important for cytogenetic investigations and diagnostics. Fluorescence in situ hybridization (FISH) is a commonly used technique for the visualization of chromosomal details. Localizing specific gene probes by FISH combined with conventional fluorescence microscopy has reached its limit. Also, microdissecting

DNA from G-banded human metaphase chromosomes by either a glass tip or by laser capture needs further improvement. Both atomic force microscopy (AFM) and scanning near-field optical microscopy (SNOM) have been used to obtain local information from G-bands and chromosomal probes (Oberringer et al 2003). The final resolution allows a more precise localization compared to standard techniques, and the extraction of very small amounts of chromosomal DNA by the scanning probe is possible. Besides new strategies towards a better G-band and fluorescent probe detection, this method is focused on the combination of biochemical and nanomanipulation techniques, which enable both nanodissection and nanoextraction of chromosomal DNA.

Applications of nanopore technology for molecular diagnostics

Nanopore technology can distinguish between and count a variety of different molecules in a complex mixture. For example, it can distinguish between hybridized or unhybridized unknown RNA and DNA molecules that differ only by a single nucleotide.

Nanopore blockade can be used to measure polynucleotide length. With further improvements, the method could in principle provide direct, high-speed detection of the sequence of bases in single molecules of DNA or RNA. Biosensor elements that are capable of identifying individual DNA strands with single-base resolution have been described (Howorka et al 2001). Each biosensor element consists of an individual DNA oligonucleotide covalently attached within the lumen of the alpha-hemolysin (alphaHL) pore to form a "DNA-nanopore". The binding of single-stranded DNA (ssDNA) molecules to the tethered DNA strand causes changes in the ionic current flowing through a nanopore. On the basis of DNA duplex lifetimes, the DNA-nanopores are able to discriminate between individual DNA strands up to 30 nucleotides in length differing by a single base substitution. This is exemplified by the detection of a drug resistance-conferring mutation in the reverse transcriptase gene of HIV. In addition, the approach was used to sequence a complete codon in an individual DNA strand tethered to a nanopore. Recent studies on single channels reconstituted into planar lipid bilayer membranes suggest that nanometer-scale pores can be used to detect, quantify and characterize a wide range of analytes that includes small ions and single stranded DNA (Kasianowicz 2002).

This technology can also be applied to the analysis of proteins. Scientists at the US   National Institute of Standards & Technology

(Gaithersburgh, MD) believe that nanopore technology for biomolecules can be applied to cancer diagnosis. The speed and simplicity of this technology will facilitate the development of molecular diagnosis and its application to personalized medicine.

Nanopore biosensors can enable direct, microsecond-time scale nucleic acid characterization without the need for amplification, chemical modification, surface adsorption, or the binding of probes. However, routine DNA analysis and sequencing will require a robust nanopore. Solid-state nanopores could be ideal, but fabrication methods need to be improved to develop an electrically addressable array of pores with reproducible diameters in the required 10^{-9} m range. A simple method that enables efficient, not too hasty, electrophoretic translocation of DNA strand through the nanopore remains to be devised. This will require a better understanding of the factors that regulate polymer translocation through nanopore.

Nanobiotechnology for identifying SNPs

Genetic analysis based on single nucleotide polymorphisms (SNPs) has the potential to enable identification of genes associated with disease susceptibility, to facilitate improved understanding and diagnosis of those diseases, and should ultimately contribute to the provision of new therapies. To achieve this end, new technology platforms are required that can increase genotyping throughput, while simultaneously reducing costs by as much as two orders of magnitude. Development of a variety of genotyping platforms with the potential to resolve this dilemma is already well advanced through research in the field of nanobiotechnology. Novel approaches to DNA extraction and amplification have reduced the times required for these processes to seconds. Microfluidic devices enable polymorphism detection through very rapid fragment separation using capillary electrophoresis and high-performance liquid chromatography, together with mixing and transport of reagents and biomolecules in integrated systems. The potential for application of established microelectronic fabrication processes to genetic analyses systems has been demonstrated (e.g. photolithography-based in situ synthesis of oligonucleotides on microarrays). Innovative application of state-of-the-art photonics and integrated circuitry are leading to improved detection capabilities. The diversity of genotyping applications envisaged in the future, ranging from the very high-throughput requirements for drug discovery through to rapid and cheap near-patient genotype analysis, suggests that several SNP genotyping platforms will be necessary to optimally address the different niches.

A nanoscale-controlled surface of DNA microarrays, where each probe DNA strand was given ample space for the incoming target DNA, provides better SNP discrimination efficiency compared to that of the DNA microarray surface where spacing is poorly controlled (Hong et al 2005). The DNA microarray fabricated on the dendron-modified slide showed excellent discrimination efficiency in a wide range of hybridization and washing temperatures. These features are important for diagnostic DNA microarrays that require high reliability and reproducibility.

DNA-protein and -nanoparticle conjugates

Semi-synthetic conjugates composed of nucleic acids, proteins and inorganic nanoparticles have been synthesized and characterized (Niemeyer 2004). For example, self-assembled oligomeric networks consisting of streptavidin and double-stranded DNA are applicable as reagents in immunoassays. Covalent conjugates of single-stranded DNA and streptavidin are utilized as biomolecular adapters for the immobilization of biotinylated macromolecules at solid substrates via nucleic acid hybridization. This 'DNA-directed immobilization' enables reversible and site-selective functionalization of solid substrates with metal and semiconductor nanoparticles or, vice versa, for the DNA-directed functionalization of gold nanoparticles with proteins, such as immunoglobulins and enzymes. This approach is applicable for the detection of chip-immobilized antigens. Moreover, covalent DNA-protein conjugates allow for their selective positioning along single-stranded nucleic acids, and thus for the construction of nanometer-scale assemblies composed of proteins and/or nanoclusters. Examples include the fabrication of functional biometallic nanostructures from gold nanoparticles and antibodies, applicable as diagnostic tools in bioanalytics.

DNA-modified nanoparticles have been used for colorimetric SNP analysis (Ihara et al 2004). These nanospheres were prepared by anchoring amino-terminated oligodeoxynucleotides (ODNs) with carboxylates onto a colored polystyrene sphere surface through amido bonds. About 220 ODN molecules were immobilized onto a nanosphere 40 nm in diameter. Preliminary studies using the microspheres with 1 μm diameter reveal that the specificity of hybridization was retained after modification. Three kinds of differently colored (RGB, red/green/blue) nanospheres bearing unique ODNs on their surface were prepared for detecting the p53 gene. The study of fluorescence resonance energy transfer (FRET) showed that spheres R and G directly contact each other in the aggregates with the wild type. The RGB color system gave aggregates with specific colors corresponding to the added

ODN samples, wild type or mutant. In addition, in the presence of both samples, all of the spheres formed aggregates with white emission as a consequence of mixing three primary colors of light. This means that the technique should enable an allele analysis.

Cantilever arrays for molecular diagnostics

Cantilevers (Concentris) are small beams similar to those used in AFM to screen biological samples for the presence of particular genetic sequences. The surface of each cantilever is coated with DNA that can bind to one particular target sequence. On exposure of the sample to beams, the surface stress bends the beams by approximately 10 nm to indicate that the beams have found the target in the sample.

Cantilever technology complements and extends current DNA and protein microarray methods because nanomechanical detection requires no labels, optical excitation, or external probes and is rapid, highly specific, sensitive, and portable. The nanomechanical response is sensitive to the concentration of oligonucleotides in solution, and thus one can determine how much of a given biomolecule is present and active. In principle cantilever arrays also could quantify gene-expression levels of mRNA, protein–protein, drug-binding interactions, and other molecular recognition events in which physical steric factors are important. It can detect a single gene within a genome. Furthermore, fabricating thinner cantilevers will enhance the molecular sensitivity further, and integrating arrays into microfluidic channels will reduce the amount of sample required significantly. In contrast to SPR, cantilevers are not limited to metallic films, and other materials will be explored, e.g., cantilevers made from polymers. In addition to surface-stress measurements, operating cantilevers in the dynamic mode will provide information on mass changes, and current investigations will determine the sensitivity of this approach. Currently it is possible to monitor more than 1,000 cantilevers simultaneously with integrated piezoresistive readout, which in principle will allow high-throughput nanomechanical genomic analysis, proteomics, biodiagnostics, and combinatorial drug discovery.

Cantilevers in an array can be functionalized with a selection of biomolecules. Surface stress changes resulting from DNA hybridization and receptor-ligand binding can be transduced into a direct nanomechanical response of microfabricated cantilevers (Fritz et al 2000). The differential deflection of the cantilevers can provide a true molecular recognition signal despite large nonspecific responses of individual cantilevers. Hybridization of complementary oligonucleotides shows that a single base mismatch between two

12-mer oligonucleotides is clearly detectable. Similar experiments on protein A-immunoglobulin interactions demonstrate the wide-ranging applicability of nanomechanical transduction to detect biomolecular recognition. Microarrays of cantilevers have been used to detect multiple unlabeled biomolecules simultaneously at nanomolar concentrations within minutes (McKendry et al 2002). Microcantilever technology might enable multiple combined tests (such as protein and DNA) to be performed on the same disposable chip.

A specific test based on 'microcantilever' can detect prostate-specific antigen (PSA). PSA antibodies are attached to the surface of the microcantilever, which is applied to a sample containing PSA (Wu et al 2001). When PSA binds to the antibodies, a change in the surface stress on the microcantilever makes it bend enough to be detected by a laser beam. This system is able to detect clinically relevant concentrations of PSA in a background of other proteins. The technique is simpler and potentially more cost-effective than other diagnostic tests because it does not require labeling and can be performed in a single reaction. It is less prone to false positives, which are commonly caused by the nonspecific binding of other proteins to the microcantilever.

Potential applications in proteomics include devices comprising many cantilevers, each coated with a different antibody, which might be used to test a sample rapidly and simultaneously for the presence of several disease-related proteins. One application is for detection of biomarkers of myocardial infarction such as creatine kinase at point-of-care. Other future applications include detection of disease by breath analysis, e.g. presence of acetone and dimethylamine (uremia). Detection of a small number of *Salmonella enterica* bacteria is achieved due to a change in the surface stress on the silicon nitride cantilever surface in situ upon binding of bacteria (Weeks et al 2003). Scanning electron micrographs indicate that less than 25 adsorbed are required for detection.

Advantages of cantilever technology for molecular recognition

Cantilever technology has the following advantages over conventional molecular diagnostics:

- It circumvents the use of PCR.

- For DNA, it has physiological sensitivity and no labeling is required.

- In proteomics, it enables detection of multiple proteins and direct observation of proteins in diseases such as those involving the cardiovascular system.

- It enables the combination of genomics and proteomics assays.

- It is compatible with silicon technology.

- It can be integrated into microfluidic devices.

Resonance light scattering technology

Resonance light scattering (RLS) technology offers uniquely powerful signal generation and detection capabilities applicable to a wide variety of analytical bioassay formats (Yguerabide and Yguerabide 2001). RLS exploits submicroscopic metallic particles (e.g. gold and silver) of uniform diameter (in the nanometer range) which scatter incident white light to generate monochromatic colored light that appears as highly intense fluorescence Each RLS particle produces intense light scattering that can be viewed with the naked eye. Under low power microscope magnification, individual 80 nm gold particles can be readily observed. The scattering produced by these particles creates a 'halo' with an apparent one-micron diameter. As a result, one can conduct ultra-sensitive assays to define location and relative frequency of target molecules. RLS signal generation technology is up to 1,000,000 times more sensitive than current fluorescence signaling technology. Other advantages of RLS technology are that RLS signals do not require computer-enhanced imaging of data as they are so intense. Research applications of RLS technology are:

- Gene Expression. Relative gene expression studies on slide-based cDNA microarrays.

- DNA Sequencing. RLS-based DNA sequencing on sequence-by-hybridization biochips.

- Microfluidics. RLS Particles for solution-based assays in nanofluidic flow-through microarrays.

- Immunohistology. Rapid in situ localization/quantitation of proteins in tissue sections using RLS-coupled antibodies.

- Homogeneous. RLS Particles for bi-molecular, microvolume studies in solution.

Clinical Applications of RLS technology are:

- RLS Technology is being used to score SNPs for discrimination of therapeutically relevant alleles.

- RLS Technology provides ultra high-sensitivity probes for in situ hybridizations to quantitate therapeutically important DNA and RNA molecules.

- Antibody-coupled RLS Particles can deliver increased sensitivity for detection of rare analytes in diagnostic assays.

- Nanoparticle-labeled bacterial RNA generates reproducible RLS signals that are at least 50 times more intense than state-of-the-art confocal-based fluorescence signals for detection of bacterial pathogens (Francois et al 2003).

DNA nanomachines for molecular diagnostics

Manipulation of DNA, by attaching a tiny radio antenna to it, can be to perform computational operations (Hamad-Schifferli et al 2002). When a radio-frequency magnetic field is transmitted to the antenna, the DNA molecule is zapped with energy and responds. The antenna is a cluster of metal, less than 100 atoms in size and about 1 nanometer long. A radio signal sent to a piece of double-stranded DNA has been shown to unwind the two strands – a process called "dehybridization." The switching is reversible, and does not affect neighboring molecules. The technique should also work on proteins, peptides and other large molecules. Applications of this technology relevant to molecular diagnostics include biomolecular detectors for homogeneous assays and direct electronic readout of biomolecular interactions

Nanobarcodes technology

Nanobarcodes with striping metallic patterns

Nanobarcodes are submicrometer metallic barcodes with striping patterns prepared by sequential electrochemical deposition of metal ions (Nicewarner-Pena et al 2001). The differential reflectivity of adjacent stripes enables identification of the striping patterns by conventional light microscopy. This readout mechanism does not interfere with the use of fluorescence for detection of analytes bound to particles by affinity capture, as demonstrated by DNA and protein bioassays. Among other applications such as SNP mapping and multiplexed assays for proteomics, Nanobarcodes can be used for population diagnostics and in point-of-care hand-held devices. This technology will enable biomarker-based drug development as a basis for personalized medicines. technology is in further development at its spinoff – Nanoplex Technologies Inc. Key performance advantages relative to existing encoded bead technologies include:

- The ability to use the widely installed base of optical microscopes for readout.

- The ability to use multiple colors of fluorophores for quantitation.

- The ability to generate hundreds to thousands of unique codes that can be distinguished at high speed.

Nanobarcodes, with various submicrometer striping patterns, may be readily distinguished in an optical microscope (Walton et al 2002). Results from a library of these particles, of which over 100 different striping patterns have been produced, reveal that more than 70 patterns may be identified with greater than 90% accuracy. The ability to chemically modify the surface of these particles makes them useful for bioanalytical measurements. Improvements in manufacturing and identification processes will lead to both larger numbers of striping patterns and improved identification accuracy.

Bio-barcode assay for proteins

An ultrasensitive method for detecting protein analytes is based on magnetic microparticle probes with antibodies for specifically binding a target of interest and nanoparticle probes that are encoded with DNA, which is unique to the protein target of interest and antibodies (Nam et al 2003). Magnetic separation of the complexed probes and target followed by dehybridization of the oligonucleotides on the nanoparticle probe surface allows the determination of the presence of the target protein by identifying the oligonucleotide sequence released from the nanoparticle probe. Because the nanoparticle probe carries with it a large number of oligonucleotides per protein binding event, there is substantial amplification and PSA can be detected at 30 attomolar concentration. Alternatively, a PCR on the oligonucleotide bar codes can boost the sensitivity to 3 attomolar. Comparable clinically accepted conventional assays for detecting the same target have sensitivity limits of 3 picomolar, six orders of magnitude less sensitive than what is observed with this method. Further development of this technology has resulted in a bio-bar-code assay with a 500 zeptomolar target DNA sensitivity limit (Nam et al 2004). Magnetic separation and subsequent release of bar code DNA from the gold nanoparticles leads to a number of bar-code DNA strands for every target DNA (see Figure 3-1). One reagent is a gold nanoparticle only 30 nm in diameter; the other is a 1-µm magnetic microparticle (MMP). During the assay, the two spheres capture and sandwich the analytes. The MMPs and whatever is bound to them are then captured using a magnet, and unreacted gold NPs are washed away. Thus, only those gold spheres that have captured the analyte remain. Each gold bead also bears an abundance of bio-barcodes, custom oligonucleotides that uniquely identify the reaction. The system ultimately detects barcodes released from the beads by heating to 55°C and not the analytes themselves. Chip-based bar code DNA detection can be done with PCR-like sensitivity but without the use of PCR.

A nanoparticle-based bio-barcode assay was used to measure the concentration of amyloidβ-derived diffusible ligands (ADDLs) in the cerebrospinal fluid (CSF) as a biomarker for Alzheimer's disease (Georganopoulou et al 2005). Commercial enzyme-linked immunoassays (ELISA) can only detect ADDLs in brain tissue where the biomarker is most highly concentrated. Studies of ADDLs in the CSF have not been possible because of their low concentration.

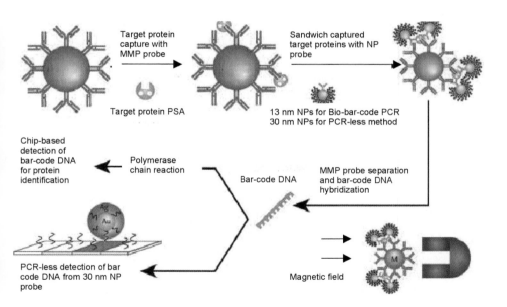

Figure 3-1: Scheme of bio-barcode assay

The protein to be detected (in this case, prostate specific antigen, PSA) is sandwiched between a magnetic microparticle (MMP) and a gold nanoparticle (NP). The MMPs and whatever is bound to them are then harvested using a magnet, and unreacted gold NPs are washed away. Thus, only those gold spheres that have captured the analyte remain. The procedure can be done with without PCR as well as with PCR (source Nam et al 2004).

The bio-barcode amplification technology, which is a million times more sensitive than ELISA, can detect ADDLs in the CSF where the biomarker is present in very low concentrations. This study is a step toward a diagnostic tool, based on soluble pathogenic markers for Alzheimer's disease. The goal is to ultimately detect and validate the marker in blood.

Using the Verigene ID system (Nanosphere Inc), one can quantify the barcodes using the kind of technology found in a flatbed scanner, providing results as clear as an at-home pregnancy strip test. Bio-bar-code system is extremely sensitive for protein detection. At 30 attomolar, it is five orders of magnitude more sensitive than is ELISA (peak sensitivity of around 3 picomolar). The system has enormous potential for multiplexing. It could hypothetically test for 415 different analytes simultaneously by tagging the different gold beads with different barcode sequences. The assay, however, the fundamental issues with antibodies, such as cross-reactivity, nonspecific binding, and lot-to-lot variability remain. Antibodies can distort, fall apart, or cling to the wrong analyte. The technology still needs further development and commercialization is anticipated.

Nanoparticle-based colorimetric DNA detection method

Nucleic acid diagnostics is dominated by fluorescence-based assays that use complex and expensive enzyme-based target or signal-amplification procedures. Many clinical diagnostic applications will require simpler, inexpensive assays that can be done in a screening mode. A 'spot-and-read' colorimetric detection method for identifying nucleic acid sequences is based on the distance-dependent optical properties of gold nanoparticles without the need for conventional signal or target amplification (Storhoff et al 2004). In this assay, nucleic acid targets are recognized by DNA-modified gold probes, which undergo a color change that is visually detectable when the solutions are spotted onto an illuminated glass waveguide. They have improved the sensitivity of the spot test by developing method that monitors scattered light rather than reflected light from 40- to 50-nm diameter gold particles. This scatter-based method enables detection of zeptomole quantities of nucleic acid targets without target or signal amplification when coupled to an improved hybridization method that facilitates probe-target binding in a homogeneous format. In comparison to a previously reported absorbance-based method, this method increases detection sensitivity by over four orders of magnitude and has been applied to the rapid detection of mecA in methicillin-resistant *Staphylococcus aureus* genomic DNA samples.

Nanosphere Inc launched its Verigene™ platform, an optical detection system, in 2003 for research environments. This device was later automated to enable one-step processing and the system includes sample preparation (for blood), microfluidics and detection technologies in an integrated system, using simple disposable cartridges. The Phase III system will be designed for medical professionals that do not typically use diagnostic systems.

SNP genotyping with gold nanoparticle probes

ClearRead™ (Nanosphere Inc), a nanoparticle technology, enables microarray-based multiplex SNP genotyping of human genomic DNA without the need for target amplification (Bao et al 2005). This direct SNP genotyping method requires no enzymes and relies on the high sensitivity of the gold nanoparticle probes. ClearRead™ technology sandwiches a target DNA SNP segment between two oligonucleotide sequences to greatly increase detection specificity and sensitivity. One segment identifies any mutations in the DNA and the probe, a highly sensitive gold nanoparticle, creates a strong signal accurately indicating the presence of a specific target SNP. Proof of principle, reproducibility, and the robust, simple and rapid characteristics of this technology were demonstrated with unamplified DNA samples representing all possible forms of three genes implicated in hypercoagulation disorders. The assay format is simple, rapid and robust pointing to its suitability for multiplex SNP profiling at the point of care.

Nanoparticle-based Up-converting Phosphor Technology

Up-Converting Phosphor Technology (UPT™) is a proprietary label detection platform technology of OraSure Technologies Inc that can be applied to the detection of minute quantities of various substances such as antigens, proteins, and DNA. UPT particles are small ceramic nanospheres composed of rare earth metals and have been shown to be 1000 times more sensitive than current fluorescent technologies. The use of OraSure's particle-based detection provides a stronger signal for each event detected and thereby enhances sensitivity in diagnostic assay systems. UPT has potential in a broad array of DNA testing applications including drug discovery, SNP analysis, and infectious disease testing. It is possible to detect nucleic acid targets in nonamplified DNA samples using easy, inexpensive, amplification-free hybridization-based assays and the ultra sensitive UPT reporters (Zuiderwijk et al 2003). Employment of UPT allows to by-pass target amplification and therefore brings genetic-based testing a step closer to the point-of-care environment. Detection of *S. pneumoniae* with only 1 ng of DNA indicates a potential for applications in the field of infectious diseases.

Surface-Enhanced Resonant Raman Spectroscopy

SERRS (Surface-Enhanced Resonant Raman Spectroscopy)-Beads (Oxonica) brings various components of the technology into a single robust nano-sized polymer-bead support with broad applications in molecular and immunodiagnostics. Focusing on organic fluorescent dyes, because of their strong excitation cross-section, compounds are selected experimentally for strong affinity for the silver enhancing surfaces and good spectral resolution. Initially using four dyes, the possibilities for tens to hundreds of unique labels is currently under development. The chosen dyes also have excitation peaks that overlap with the metal plasmon frequency, thereby adding the all-important resonant amplification to the signal intensity.

At the core of the bead is the Raman-active substrate, where silver colloid, with defined physical characteristics, provides the surface-enhancement substrate and is combined with the dye or dyes for specific bead encoding. Control of the various parameters surrounding dye:colloid aggregate permits SERRS response to be modulated as desired.

To protect the SERRS-active complex from degradation, the aggregate is encapsulated in a polymer coating, a process that incorporates a multitude of dye:colloid particles into the same bead. This leads to highly sensitive beads with responses in excess of that achieved using the conformation of a single dye molecules on an enhancing surface.

The polymer coating is treated further with a polymer shell to allow a variety of biologically relevant probe molecules (e.g. antibodies, antigens, nucleic acids) to be attached through standard bioconjugation techniques.

Oxonica is working closely with Avalon Instruments to develop its RamanSpec plate reader with the SERRS-Beads configuration. While current development is focused on heterogeneous assays in a 96-well assay sample presentation, other designs include higher plate capacities (384-well) for higher throughput screening and microarray slide reading for DNA and proteomic analysis.

Enhancement of Raman signal near silver colloidal nanoparticles is exploited to study the Raman spectrum of yeast cytochrome c (YCc) from *Saccharomyces cerevisiae* in a single-molecule (Delfino et al 2005). The investigation is performed on proteins both in solution and immobilized onto a glass slide using a quasiresonant laser line as exciting source with low excitation intensity. In both cases, spectra acquired at different times exhibit dramatic temporal fluctuations in both the total spectrum and in the specific line intensity, even though averaging of several individual spectra reproduces the main Raman features of bulk YCc. Analysis of the spectral intensity fluctuations from solutions reveals a multimodal distribution of some specific Raman lines, consistent with the approaching of single molecule regime. Among other results, the statistical analysis of the spectra from immobilized samples seems to indicate dynamical processes involving the reorientation of the heme with respect to the metal surface.

Near-infrared (NIR)-emissive polymersomes

Fluorescent materials called porphyrins have been lodged within the surface of a polymersome, a cell-like vesicle, to image a tumor in a living rodent (Ghoroghchian et al 2005). Near-infrared (NIR)-emissive polymersomes (50 nm to 50μm-diameter polymer vesicles) were generated through cooperative self assembly of amphiphilic diblock copolymers and conjugated multi(porphyrin)-based NIR fluorophores (NIRFs). When compared with natural vesicles comprised of phospholipids, polymersomes were uniquely capable of incorporating and uniformly distributing numerous large hydrophobic NIRFs exclusively in their lamellar membranes. Within these sequestered compartments, long polymer chains regulate the mean fluorophore-fluorophore interspatial separation as well as the fluorophore-localized electronic environment. Porphyrin-based NIRFs manifest photophysical properties within the polymersomal matrix akin to those established for these high-emission dipole strength fluorophores in organic solvents, thereby yielding uniquely emissive vesicles. Furthermore, the total fluorescence emanating from the assemblies gives rise to a localized optical signal of sufficient intensity to penetrate through the dense tumor tissue of a live animal. Robust NIR-emissive polymersomes thus define a soft matter platform with exceptional potential to facilitate deep-tissue fluorescence-based imaging for in vivo diagnostic and drug-delivery applications.

Nanobiotechnology for detection of proteins

Detection of proteins is an important part of molecular diagnostics. Uses of protein nanobiochips and nano-barcode technology for detection of proteins will be described in Chapter 4. Other methods will be included in this section.

Nanoscale protein analysis

Most current protocols including protein purification/ display and automated identification schemes yield unacceptably low recoveries, thus limiting the overall process in terms of sensitivity and speed and require more starting material. Low abundant proteins and proteins that can only be isolated from limited source material (e.g., biopsies) can be subjected to nanoscale protein analysis – nano-capture of specific proteins and complexes, and optimization of all subsequent sample handling steps leading to mass analysis of peptide fragments. This is a focused approach, also termed targeted proteomics, and involves examination of subsets of the proteome, e.g., those proteins that are either specifically modified, or bind to a particular DNA sequence, or exist as members of higher order complexes, or any combination thereof. This approach is used at Memorial Sloan-Kettering Cancer Center and Cornell University, New York, to identify how genetic determinants of cancer alter cellular physiology and response to agonists.

Multi Photon Detection

A new detection technique called Multi Photon Detection (MPD) is in development at BioTrace Inc and enables quantitation of sub-zeptomole amounts of proteins. It will be used for diagnostic proteomics, particularly for cytokines and other low abundance proteins. BioTrace is developing supersensitive protein biochips to detect as low as 5 fg/ml (0.2 attomole/ml) concentration of proteins. Thus, this innovative type of the P-chips might permit about 1,000 fold better sensitivity than current protein biochips.

Nanoflow liquid chromatography

The use of liquid chromatography (LC) in analytical chemistry is well established but relatively low sensitivity associated with conventional LC makes it unsuitable for the analysis of certain biological samples. Furthermore, the flow rates at which it is operated are not compatible with the use of specific detectors, such as electrospray ionization mass spectrometers. Therefore, due to the analytical demands of biological samples, miniaturized LC techniques were developed to allow for the analysis of samples with greater sensitivity than that afforded by conventional LC. In nanoflow LC (nanoLC) chromatographic separations are performed using flow rates in the range of low nanoliter per minute, which result in high analytical sensitivity due to the large concentration efficiency afforded by this type of chromatography. NanoLC, in combination to tandem mass spectrometry, was first used to analyze peptides and as an alternative to other mass spectrometric methods to identify gel-separated proteins. Gel-free analytical approaches based on LC and nanoLC separations have been developed, which are allowing proteomics to be performed in faster and more comprehensive manner than by using strategies based on the classical 2D gel electrophoresis approaches (Cutillas 2005).

Protein identification using nanoflow liquid chromatography-mass spectrometry (MS)-MS (LC-MS-MS) provides reliable sequencing information for low femtomole level of protein digests. However, this task is more challenging for subfemtomole peptide levels.

High-field asymmetric waveform ion mobility mass spectrometry

An ion mobility technology - high-field asymmetric waveform ion mobility mass spectrometry (FAIMS) has been introduced as online ion selection methods compatible with electrospray ionization (ESI). FAIMS uses ion separation to improve detection limits of peptide ions when used in conjunction with electrospray and nanoelectrospray MS. This facilitates the identification of low-abundance peptide ions often present at ppm levels in complex proteolytic digests and expand the sensitivity and selectivity of nanoLC–MS analyses in global and targeted proteomics approaches. This functionality likely will play an important role in drug discovery and biomarker programs for monitoring of disease progression and drug efficacy (Venne et al 2005).

Captamers with proximity extension assay for proteins

Multivalent circular aptamers or 'captamers' are formed through the merger of aptameric recognition functions with the DNA as a nanoscale scaffold. Aptamers are useful as protein-binding motifs for diagnostic applications, where their ease of discovery, thermal stability and low cost make them ideal components for incorporation into targeted protein assays. Captamers are compatibile with a highly

93

sensitive protein detection method termed the 'proximity extension' assay (Di Giusto et al 2004). The circular DNA architecture facilitates the integration of multiple functional elements into a single molecule: aptameric target recognition, nucleic acid hybridization specificity and rolling circle amplification. Successful exploitation of these properties is demonstrated for the molecular analysis of thrombin, with the assay delivering a detection limit nearly three orders of magnitude below the dissociation constants of the two contributing aptamer-thrombin interactions. Real-time signal amplification, detection under isothermal conditions, specificity and sensitivity would suggest potential application as a protein assay required for the further development of personalized medicine.

4. NANOBIOCHIPS/ NANOARRAYS FOR MOLECULAR DIAGNOSTICS

Abstract

This chapter is devoted to nanobiochips and nanoarrays that are the next stage of continuing miniaturization after microfluidics. Dip pen nanolithography (DPN) uses the tip of an AFM to write molecular "inks" directly on a surface. Biomolecules such as proteins and viruses can be positioned on surfaces to form nanoarrays that retain their biological activity. Nanobiotechnology has been applied to protein biochips as well resulting in a variety of protein nanochips.

Introduction

The trend towards miniaturization initially focused on devices that contained micrometer-sized features designed for a particular analytical purpose, e.g. biochips. Now, the focus is shifting to analytical applications based on nanosized objects such as nanotubes, nanochannels, nanoparticles and nanopores. These nanofabricated objects provide new tools for molecular diagnostics. Because of the small dimension, most of the applications of nanobiotechnology in molecular diagnostics still fall under the broad category of biochips/ microarrays but are more correctly termed nanochips and nanoarrays. Nanotechnology-on-a-chip is a general description that can be applied to several methods. Some of these do not use nanotechnologies but merely have the capability to analyze nanoliter amounts of fluids.

Biochips, constructed with microelectromechanical systems on a micron scale, are related to micromanipulation, whereas nanotechnology-based chips on a nanoscale are related to nanomanipulation. Even though microarray/biochip methods employing the detection of specific biomolecular interactions are now an indispensable tool for molecular diagnostics, there are some limitations. DNA microarrays and ELISA rely on the labeling of samples with a fluorescent or radioactive tag - a highly sensitive procedure that is time-consuming and expensive.

Micro- and nano-electromechanical systems

The rapid pace of miniaturization in the semiconductor industry has resulted in faster and more powerful computing and instrumentation, which have begun to revolutionize medical diagnosis and therapy. Some of the instrumentation used for nanotechnology is an extension of MEMS (Micro ElectroMechanical Systems), which refers to a key enabling technology used to produce micro-fabricated sensors and systems. The potential mass application of MEMS lies in the fact that miniature components are batch fabricated using the manufacturing techniques developed in the semiconductor microelectronics industry enabling miniaturized, low-cost, high-performance and integrated electromechanical systems. The "science of miniaturization" is a much more appropriate name than MEMS and it involves a good understanding of scaling laws, different manufacturing methods and materials that are being applied in nanotechnology.

MEMS devices currently range in size from one to hundreds of micrometers and can be as simple as the singly supported cantilever beams used in AFM or as complicated as a video projector with thousands of electronically controllable microscopic mirrors. NEMS devices exist correspondingly in the nanometer realm – nano-electromechanical systems (NEMS). The concept of using externally controllable MEMS devices to measure and manipulate biological matter (BioMEMS) on the cellular and subcellular levels has attracted much attention recently. This is because initial work has shown the ability to detect single base pair mismatches of DNA and to quantifiably detect antigens using cantilever systems. In addition is the ability to controllably grab and manipulate individual cells and subsequently release them unharmed.

BioMEMS

Because BioMEMS involves the interface of MEMS with biological environments, the biological components are crucially important. To date, they have mainly been nucleic acids, antibodies and receptors that are involved in passive aspects of detection and measurement. These molecules retain their biological activity following chemical attachment to the surfaces of MEMS structures (most commonly, thiol groups to gold) and their interactions are monitored through mechanical (deflection of a cantilever), electrical (change in voltage or current in the sensor) or optical (surface plasmon resonance) measurements. The biological components are in the nanometer range or smaller; therefore, the size of these systems is limited by the minimum feature sizes achievable using the fabrication techniques of the inorganic structures, currently 100 nm to 1 μm. Commercially available products resulting from further miniaturization could be problematic because of the expanding cost and complexity of optical lithography equipment and the inherent slowness of electron beam techniques. In addition to size limitations, the effects of friction have plagued multiple moving parts in inorganic MEMS, limiting device speeds and useful lifetimes (Schmidt and Montemagno 2002).

Microarrays and nanoarrays

Macroarraying (or gridding) is a macroscopic scheme of organizing colonies or DNA into arrays on large nylon filters ready for screening by hybridization. In microarrays, however, the sample spot sizes are usually less than 200 microns in diameter and require microscopic analysis. Microarrays have sample or ligand molecules (e.g., antibodies) at fixed locations on the chip while microfluidics involves the transport of material, samples, and/or reagents on the chip.

Microarrays provide a powerful way to analyze the expression of thousands of genes simultaneously. Genomic arrays are an important tool in medical diagnostic and pharmaceutical research. They have an impact on all phases of the drug discovery process from target identification through differential gene expression, identification and screening of small molecule candidates, to toxicogenomic studies for drug safety. To meet the increasing needs, the density and information content of the microarrays is being improved. One approach is fabrication of chips with smaller, more closely packed features - ultrahigh density arrays, which will yield:

- High information content by reduction of feature size from 200μm to 50 nm

- Reduction in sample size

- Improved assay sensitivity

Nanoarrays are the next stage in the evolution of miniaturization of microarrays. Whereas microarrays are prepared by robotic spotting or optical lithography, limiting the smallest size to several microns, nanoarrays require further developments in lithography strategies. Technologies available include the following:

- Electron beam lithography

- Dip-pen nanolithography

- Scanning probe lithography

- Finely focused ion beam lithography

- Nano-imprint lithography

Dip Pen Nanolithography for nanoarrays

Dip Pen Nanolithography™ (DPN™) commercialized by NanoInk Inc employs uses the tip of an AFM to write molecular "inks" directly on a surface. Biomolecules such as proteins and viruses can be positioned on surfaces to form nanoarrays that retain their biological activity. DPN is schematically depicted in Figure 4-1.

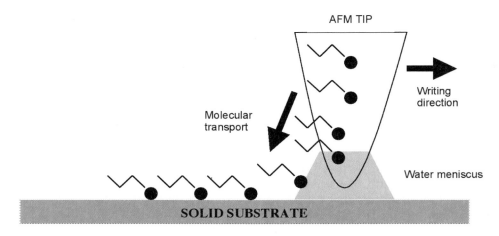

Figure 4-1: Schematic representation of Dip Pen Nanolithography (DPN)

Advantages of DPN are as follows:

Ultrahigh resolution. DPN is capable of producing structures with line widths of less than 15 nanometers. This is compared to photolithography, which supports features of no less than 65 nm line width, and slower e-beam and laser lithography systems, which support features of 15 nm line width.

Flexibility. Direct fabrication is possible with many substances, from biomolecules to metals.

Accuracy. By leveraging existing highly accurate atomic force microscopy technology, DPN utilizes the best possible means for determining exactly where features are being placed on the substrate. This allows for the integration of multiple component nanostructures and for immediate inspection and characterization of fabricated structures.

Low capital cost. Techniques such as e-beam lithography that approach DPN-scale resolution are considerably more expensive to purchase, operate and maintain.

Ease of use. DPN systems may be operated by non-specialized personnel with minimal training. Further, DPN may be performed under normal ambient laboratory conditions with humidity control.

Speed. 100-nm spots can be deposited with a single DPN pen in less than a second. DPN can be used to fabricate arrays of a single molecule with more than 100,000 spots over 100 x 100 micron in less than an hour.

Protein nanoarrays

High-throughput protein arrays allow the miniaturized and parallel analysis of large numbers of diagnostic markers in complex samples. This capability can be enhanced by nanotechnology. DPN technique has been extended to protein arrays with features as small as 45 nm and immunoproteins as well as enzymes can be deposited. Selective binding of antibodies to protein nanoarrays can be detected without the use of labels by monitoring small (5-15 nm) topographical height increases in AFM images.

BioForce Nanosciences' Protein Nanoarrays contain up to 25 million spots per sq cm. They can be used to detect protein-protein interactions. BioForce's NanoReader uses a customized AFM to decipher molecules on a NanoArray chip.

Microfluidics and nanofluidics

Microfluidics is the handling and dealing with small quantities (e.g. microliters, nanoliters or even picoliters) of fluids flowing in channels the size of a human hair (approx 50 microns thick) even narrower. Fluids in this environment show very different properties than in the macro world. This new field of technology was enabled by advances in microfabrication – the etching of silicon to create very small features. Microfluidics is one of the most important innovations of biochip technology. Typical dimensions of microfluidic chips are 1 - 50 cm^2 and have channels 5 - 100 microns. Usual volumes are 0.01 - 10 microliters but can be less. Microfluidics is the link between microarrays and nanoarrays as we reduce the dimensions and volumes.

Microfluidics is the underlying principle of lab-on-a-chip devices, which carry out complex analyses, while reducing sample and chemical consumption, decreasing waste and improving precision and efficiency. The idea is to be able to squirt a very small sample into the chip, push a button and the chip will do all the work, delivering a report at the end. Microfluidics allows the reduction in size with a corresponding increase in the throughput of handling, processing and analyzing the sample. Other advantages of microfluidics include increased reaction rates, enhanced detection sensitivity and control of adverse events.

Drawbacks and limitations of microfluidics and designing of microfluidic chips include the following:

- Difficulties in microfluidic connections

- Because of laminar flows, mixing can only be performed by diffusion

- Large capillary forces

- Clogging

- Possible evaporation and drying up of the sample

Applications of microfluidics include the following:

- DNA analysis

- Protein analysis

- Gene expression and differential display analysis

- Biochemical analysis

Nanotechnology on a chip

Nanotechnology on a chip is a new paradigm for total chemical analysis systems (Jain 2005d). The ability to make chemical and biological information much cheaper and easier to obtain is expected to fundamentally change healthcare, food safety and law enforcement. Lab-on-a-chip technology involves micro-total analysis systems that are distinguished from simple sensors because they conduct a complete analysis; a raw mixture of chemicals goes in and an answer comes out. Hand-held lab-on-a-chips are in development to detect air-borne chemical warfare agents and liquid-based explosives agents. This development project brings together an interdisciplinary team with areas of expertise including microfabrication, chemical sensing, microfluidics, and bioinformatics. Although nanotechnology plays an important role in current efforts, miniaturized versions of conventional architecture and components such as valves, pipes, pumps, separation columns, are patterned after their macroscopic counterparts. Nanotechnology will provide the ability to build materials with switchable molecular functions could provide completely new approaches to valves, pumps, chemical separations, and detection. For example, fluid streams could be directed by controlling surface energy without the need for a predetermined architecture of physical channels. Switchable molecular membranes and the like could replace mechanical valves. By eliminating the need for complex fluidic networks and micro-scale components used in current approaches, a fundamentally new approach will allow greater function in much smaller, lower power total chemical analysis systems.

A new scheme for the detection of molecular interactions based on optical readout of nanoparticle labels has been developed. Capture DNA probes were arrayed on a glass chip and incubated with nanoparticle-labeled target DNA probes, containing a complementary sequence. Binding events were monitored by optical means, using reflected and transmitted light for the detection of surface-bound nanoparticles. Control experiments exclude significant influence of nonspecific binding on the observed contrast. Scanning force microscopy revealed the distribution of nanoparticles on the chip surface (Reichert et al 2000).

BioForce Nanosciences has taken the technology of the microarray to the next level by creating the "nanoarray," an ultra-miniaturized version of the traditional microarray that can actually measure interactions between individual molecules down to resolutions of as little as one nanometer. Here, 400 nanoarray spots can be placed in the same area as a traditional microarray spot (see Figure 4-2). Nanoarrays are the next evolutionary step in the miniaturization of bioaffinity tests for proteins, nucleic acids, and receptor-ligand pairs. On a BioForce NanoArrayT, as many as 1,500 different samples can be queried in the same area now needed for just one domain on a traditional microarray.

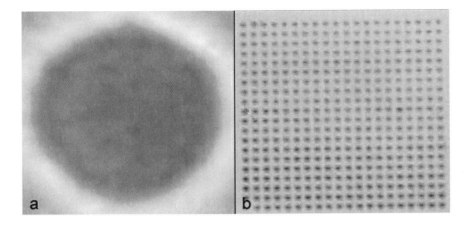

Figure 4-2: Nanoarrrays versus microarrays

400 spots can be placed on the same area of a nanoarray (b) as that required for a microarray (a). Photo courtesy of BioForce Nanosciences.

Microfluidic chips for nanoliter volumes

Nanoliter implies extreme reduction in quantity of fluid analyte in a microchip. The use of the word "nano" in nanoliter (nl) is in a different dimension than in nanoparticle, which is in nanometer (nm) scale. Diagnostic Companies with "nano" in their name that may have other technologies. For example, Nanolytics Inc with lab-on-chip based on nanoliter microfluidics and Nanogen with NanoChip based on microelectronics.

In another technique, chemical compounds within individual nanoliter droplets of glycerol were microarrayed on to glass slides at 400 spots/cm^2 (Gosalia and Diamond 2003). Using aerosol deposition, subsequent reagents and water were metered into each reaction center to rapidly assemble diverse multicomponent reactions without cross contamination or the need for surface linkage. This proteomics technique allowed the kinetic profiling of protease mixtures, protease-substrate interactions, and high-throughput screening reactions. From one printing run that consumes <1 nanomole of each compound, large combinatorial libraries can be subjected to numerous separation-free homogeneous assays at volumes 103-104 smaller than current high-throughput methods. The rapid assembly of thousands of nanoliter reactions per slide using a small biological sample (2 ml) represents a new functional proteomics format implemented with standard microarraying and spot-analysis tools. Currently available nanoliter/biochip technologies are shown in Table 4-1.

Table 4-1: Nanoliter/biochip technologies for molecular diagnostics

Technology	Company/Laboratory	Applications
Microagitation chips: nanopumps can move nanoliter droplets to control mixing and subsequent chemical reactions	Advalytix AG (Brunnthal, Germany)	To make DNA/protein microarrays a reliable tool for high throughput diagnostic applications
RNA 6000 Nano LabChip kit	Agilent Technologies / Caliper (Palo Alto, CA)	For the automated quality control of total and messenger RNA
The nanofluidic Living™ Chip for massively parallel and low-volume analysis	BioTrove Inc (Woburn, MA)	SNP genotyping
LabChip and Sciclone® liquid handler platform handle volumes in nanoliter range	Caliper Life Sciences (Hopkinton, MA)	Molecular diagnostics
Chip with internally generated pressure to propel nanoliter liquid plugs through a micro-channel network	HandyLab Inc (Ann Arbor, Michigan)	For point-of-care diagnosis of infectious diseases
NanoJet technology performs a liquid jet by means of a microvalve, which directly switches the jet on and off volumes of 50nl	Microdrop GmbH (Norderstedt, Germany)	With 100 spots on one chip, 100 diagnostic tests are possible with only one small drop of blood
Microfluidics- and nanofluidics-based systems	Micronics Inc (Redmond, WA)	Clinical laboratory diagnostics and analytical chemical determinations
NanoChip Molecular Biology Workstation to bridge research and clinical diagnostics	Nanogen Inc (San Diego, CA)	To provide quick and accurate analysis of DNA, RNA and proteins
Electrowetting: rapid and reversible control of contact angle between a surface and an electrolyte droplet by applying electric field	Nanolytics Inc (Raleigh, NC)	To handle nanoliter and subnanoliter fluid volumes on biochip assays
Micro parallel liquid chromatography using nanoliters of sample materials	Nanostream Inc (Pasadena, CA)	DNA sequencing and clinical diagnostics
Nanostructured surfaces for nanofluidic bioanalytics	SuNyx (Cologne, Germany)	Analytic biochips
Microplate Differential Calorimetry: detection of temperature changes in volumes ranging from 10 nl to 10ml	Vivactis (Leuven, Belgium)	Diagnostics

NanoChip

NanoChip (Nanogen Inc) is a microelectronic chip format suitable for rapid single nucleotide polymorphism (SNP) analysis and genetic dissection of complex phenotypes. In beta testing, the NanoChip system has been shown to provide accuracy equal to or better than DNA sequencing and other methods for SNP confirmation. Unlike other systems, the NanoChip system uses electronically accelerated hybridization under very low salt conditions, potentially avoiding problems with DNA conformation and secondary structures, whereas most sequencing and primer extension technologies require high salt conditions. The NanoChip system allows the user to array and analyze DNA on its NanoChip cartridges in user-selected formats in a single day with walk-away automation. The NanoChip system integrates advanced microelectronics and molecular biology into a platform technology with broad commercial applications in the fields of biomedical research, genomics, medical diagnostics, genetic testing and drug discovery.

A SNP typing protocol has been developed for the NanoChip (Borsting et al 2005). An electric currenct can be applied to one, several, or all electrodes at the same time according to a loading protocol generated by the user. Biotinylated DNA is directed to the pad(s) via the electronic field(s) and bound to streptavidin in the hydrogel layer. Subsequently, fluorescently labeled reporter oligos and a stabilizer oligo are hybridized to the bound DNA. Base stacking between the short reporter and the longer stabilizer oligo stabilizes the binding of a matching reporter, whereas the binding of a reporter carrying a mismatch in the SNP position will be relatively weak. Thermal stringency is applied to the NanoChip array according to a reader protocol generated by the user and the fluorescent label on the matching reporter is detected.

A matrix analysis was performed for different bacterial species and complementary capture probes on NanoChip to optimize detection of hybridization signals for bacterial detection (Barlaan et al 2005). Results showed that, when using the longer amplicon, not all bacterial targets hybridized with the complementary capture probes, which was characterized by the presence of false-positive signals. However, with the shorter amplicons, all bacterial species were correctly and completely detected using the constructed complementary capture probes.

The NanoChip system has been used for subtyping human immunodeficiency virus type 1 (HIV-1) strains using probes complementary to the V1 region of the env gene. Overall, the NanoChip assay produced results comparable to those for heteroduplex mobility assay and sequencing and provides a convenient and cost-effective means by which to subtype HIV-1 (Saunders et al 2005).

Use of nanotechnology in microfluidics

Construction of nanofluidic channels

Techniques such as nanoimprinting are used to construct large arrays of nanoscale grooves with efficiency and speed. Now such grooves can be sealed with similar ease, to form nanofluidic channels. Laser-assisted direct imprint technique enables construction of millions of enclosed nanofluidic channels side by side on a single substrate, which is ideal for such parallel processing. By sputter-depositing silicon dioxide at an angle on to an array of prefabricated nanochannels imprinted into the surface of a biopolymer substrate, not only is an effective and uniform seal formed over the entire array, but the channels are further narrowed down to 10 nm, from an initial width of 55 nm. This process could be easily used for narrowing and sealing micro- and nano-fluidic structures formed by other patterning techniques. By minimizing the hollow space in such structures, it could help surpass existing limitations in the spatial resolution of these techniques.

A chip-scale maze for combing out strands of DNA and inserting them into nanoscale channels was made using standard, inexpensive lithographic techniques (Cao et al 2002a). Their 'gradient nanostructure' might be used to isolate and stretch DNA molecules for analysis, e.g., to look for bound proteins such as transcription factors along the strand. Such molecules would be obscured in normal solution because DNA, like any other linear polymer, collapses into a random coil as a featureless blob. The strands can, in principle, be straightened by feeding them into channels just a few tens of nanometers wide, using nanofluidic techniques.

Flexible tubes have been fabricated with diameters of 100 nanometers, i.e. ten times narrower than those used in today's microfluidic systems (Melechko et al 2002). The tubes could be used to make stacked, interconnected fluidic networks designed to shunt fluids around biochips that sense and analyze chemicals. The method was discovered during deposition of a certain type of polymer into tiny silicon grooves, which closed the gaps at ends forming tubes. The potential of the process to make tiny networks of tubes for use in microfluidics was realized. The method is also compatible with conventional processes for making chips and can be used to integrate the networks with electronic chip components.

Restriction mapping of DNA molecules has been performed using restriction endonucleases in nanochannels with diameters of 100-200 nm (Riehn et al 2005). Restriction mapping with endonucleases is a central method in molecular biology. It is based on the measurement of fragment lengths after digestion, while possibly maintaining the respective order. The location of the restriction reaction within the device is controlled by electrophoresis and diffusion of Mg^{2+} and EDTA. It is possible to measure the positions of restriction sites with precision using single DNA molecules with a resolution of 1.5 kbp within 1 min.

Nanoscale flow visualization

Most of the microscale flow visualization methods evolved from methods developed originally for macroscale flow. It is unlikely, however, that developed microscale flow visualization methods will be translated to nanoscale flows in a similar manner. Resolving nanoscale features with visible light presents a fundamental challenge. Although point-detection scanning methods have potential to increase the flow measurement resolution on the microscale, spatial resolution is ultimately limited by the optical probe volume (length scale on the order of 100 nm), which, in turn, is limited by the wavelength of light employed (Sinton 2004). Optical spatially resolved flow measurements in nanochannels are difficult to visualize. There is a need for refinement of microscale flow visualization methods and the development of direct flow measurement methods for nanoflows.

Moving (levitation) of nanofluidic drops with physical forces

The manipulation of droplets/particles that are isolated (levitated in gas/vacuum) from laboratory samples containing chemicals, cells, bacteria or viruses, is important both for basic research in physics, chemistry, biology, biochemistry, and colloidal science and for applications in nanotechnology and microfluidics. Various optical, electrostatic, electromagnetic and acoustic methods are used for levitation.

Microfluidic drops can be moved with light by the lotus effect (Rosario et al 2004). On a super-rough surface, when light shines on one side of a drop, the surface changes, the molecules switch and the drop moves. This technology can be used for quickly analyzing and screening small amounts of biological materials. Called digital microfluidics, this approach enables one to quickly move small drops around by shining light on them. Hundreds of screens could be done on only one particular surface. The molecules, e.g. protein traces, do not interfere with movements of the drops because the surfaces are hydrophobic and the molecules have little contact with the surface.

The size of diamagnetic levitation devices has been reduced by using micron scale permanent magnets to create a magnetic micromanipulation chip, which operates with femtodroplets levitated in air (Lyuksyutov et al 2004). The droplets used are one billion times smaller in volume than has been demonstrated by conventional methods. The levitated particles can be positioned with up to 300 nm accuracy and precisely rotated and assembled. Using this lab-on-a-chip it might be possible to do the same thing with a large number of fluids, chemicals and even red blood cells, bacteria and viruses.

Nanoarrays for molecular diagnostics

Several nanoarrays and nanobiochips are in development. Some of these will be reviewed here.

NanoPro™ System

The NanoPro™ System (BioForce Nanosciences Inc) consists of three separate components:

1. The NanoArrayer™ embodies proprietary instrumentation and methods for creating a broad spectrum of NanoArray™-based biological tests. This device places molecules at defined locations on a surface with nanometer spatial resolution. The arrays of molecules (NanoArrays™, see below) are unique to BioForce and can only be created with a NanoArrayer™.

2. NanoArrays™ are ultra-miniaturized biological tests with applications in many areas. The Company's first NanoArray™ products are presently being evaluated for commercial utilization by potential users and are targeted toward the proteomics/ genomics and diagnostics markets. These products include a custom nucleic acid NanoArray™ for RNA expression profiling as well as virus detection NanoArray™ called the ViriChip™. NanoArray™ chips are for protein expression profiling and immunodiagnostics.

3. The NanoReader™ is a customized Atomic Force Microscope (AFM) optimized for reading NanoArray™ chips. Using the AFM as a readout method optimizes analysis, with following advantages:

-   No need for secondary reporter systems such as fluorescence, radioactivity or enzyme linked detection.

- Reductions in materials used as several thousand molecules can be covered with one test.

- Increased sensitivity with single molecule detection ultimately.

Nanoparticle protein chip

A sensitive technique is being developed for optical detection of nanogold particle-labeled molecules on protein microarray by applying the surface plasmon resonance and specific molecular binding using rolling circles amplification (Hsu and Huang 2004). A new type of protein chip is being developed based on protein-binding silica-nanoparticles at the Fraunhofer Institute for Interfacial Engineering and Biotechnology IGB (Stuttgart, Germany). The surface of this minute particle with a diameter of less than 100 nm can be configured with many different capture proteins. The particles configured in this way are then applied to silicon carriers in thin, even layers. After contact is made with a sample, the chips can be analyzed using state-of-the-art mass spectrometry, MALDI-TOF mass spectrometry. Knowing the masses of the bound proteins provides a direct indication of their identity.

Protein nanobiochip

Nanotechnology Group of the NEC Corporation has developed a prototype protein analysis technology that can analyze samples about 20 times faster than conventional techniques. The company's technology can complete an analysis of a blood sample in about 60 minutes or 70 minutes, compared to the day or so such analysis takes by conventional methods.

Biomarker proteins as early warning signs for diseases such as cancer can be identified for diagnostic purposes by finding their isoelectric points and their molecular weights. Isoelectric points are chemical features that refer to the electrical state of a molecule when it has no net charge. Conventional protein chips use a gel across which an electric current is applied to find the targeted protein's isoelectric points. In the new process, instead of being filtered through a block of gel, the protein molecules are separated by their isoelectric points by a capillary action as the proteins flow in a solution along channels in the chip. A test chip by NEC measures 21 mm^2 and contained four sets of tiny channels in which the capillary action takes place. The protein molecules are then dried and irradiated by a laser. Their molecular weights are then measured by a mass spectrometer. The laser helps the proteins leave the chip, and the mass spectrometer is used to judge the molecular weights of the protein molecules in the samples by measuring how early they reach a detector. In the mass spectrometer, light molecules fly faster than heavy ones in an electric field. The mass spectrometer judges the weight of the molecules by monitoring the timing of when each molecule reaches a detector. In addition to being faster than techniques that use gel blocks, the new method also needs blood samples of about 1µL compared to about 20µL or more that are needed using gel-based techniques. NEC is now planning clinical trials, which should last between two and three years. If those trials go well, the company should commercialize the technology around or after 2008. When commercialized, the technique could be used for health checks that might cost as little as $100.

Protein biochips based on fluorescence planar wave guide technology

The fluorescence planar wave guide (PWG) technology has demonstrated exceptional performance in terms of sensitivity, making it a viable method for detection in chip-based microarrays. Thin film PWGs as used in ZeptoMARK™ protein microarrays (Zeptosens Bioanalytical Solutions) consist of a 150 to 300 nm thin film of a material with high refractive index, which is deposited on a transparent support with lower refractive index (e.g., glass or polymer). A parallel laser light beam is coupled into the waveguiding film by a diffractive grating, which is etched or embossed into the substrate. The light propagates within this film and creates a strong evanescent field perpendicular to the direction of propagation into the adjacent medium. It has been shown that the intensity of this evanescent field can be enhanced dramatically by increasing the refractive index of the waveguiding layer and equally by decreasing the layer thickness. Compared to confocal excitation the field intensity close to the surface can be increased by a factor of up to 100. The field strength decays exponentially with the distance from the waveguide surface, and its penetration depth is limited to about 400 nm. This effect can be utilized to selectively excite only fluorophores located at or near the surface of the waveguide. By taking advantage of the high field intensity and the confinement of this field to the close proximity of the waveguide PWG technology combines highly selective fluorescence detection with highest sensitivity.

For bioanalytical applications, specific capture probes or recognition elements for the analyte of interest are immobilized on the waveguide surface. The presence of the analyte in a sample applied to a PWG chip is detected using fluorescent reporter molecules attached to the analyte or one of its binding partners in the assay. Upon fluorescence excitation by the evanescent field, excitation and detection of fluorophores is restricted to the sensing surface, whilst signals from unbound molecules in the bulk solution are not detected. The result is a significant increase in the signal/noise ratio compared to conventional optical detection methods.

A variety of proteins can be immobilized on PWG microarrays as selective recognition elements for the investigation of specific ligand-protein interactions such as antigen-antibody, protein-protein and protein-DNA interactions. Protein microarrays based on PWG allow the simultaneous, qualitative and quantitative analysis of protein interactions with high sensitivity in a massively parallel manner. This method enables cost-effective determination of efficacy of drug candidates in a vast number of preclinical study samples.

5. NANOBIOSENSORS

Abstract

Biosensors incorporate a biological sensing element that converts a change in an immediate environment to signals that can be processed. Nanomaterials are exquisitely sensitive chemical and biological sensors and are used in the construction of nanobiosensors for detection of chemical as well as biological materials. Several types of nanobiosensors are described including optical biosensors that rely on the optical properties of lasers to monitor and quantify interactions of biomolecules on specially derived surfaces or biochips. Some nanobiosensors are based on surface plasmon resonance (SPR), which is an optical-electrical phenomenon involving the interaction of light with the electrons of a metal.

Introduction

Biosensors incorporate a biological sensing element that converts a change in an immediate environment to signals that can be processed. Biosensors have been implemented for a number of applications ranging from environmental pollutant detection to defense monitoring. Biosensors have two intriguing characteristics: (1) they have a naturally evolved selectivity to biological or biologically active analytes; and (2) biosensors have the capacity to respond to analytes in a physiologically relevant manner. Molecular biosensors are based on antibodies, enzymes, ion channels, or nucleic acids (Jain 2003b). In theory, nucleic acid analysis provides a higher degree of certainty than traditional antibody technologies because antibodies occasionally exhibit cross reactivity with antigens other than the analyte of interest. In practice, however, development of nucleic acid sensor systems has been hampered by the challenges presented in sample preparation. Nucleic acid isolation remains the rate-limiting step for all of the state-of-the-art molecular analyses. The basic principle of a biosensor is shown in Figure 5-1.

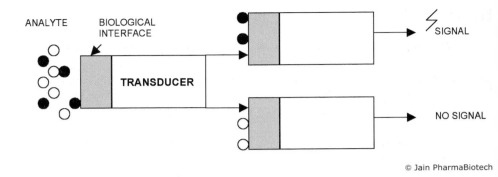

Figure 5-1: Basic principle of a biosensor

The compound of interest (black circles) in a mixture of substances specifically interacts with the biological part of the sensor. The resulting biological signal is converted into a physical signal (e.g., electric or optical) by a transducer. Substances, which are not capable of interacting with the biological component (hollow circles), will not produce any signal.

Nanosensors are devices that employ nanomaterials, exploiting novel size-dependent properties, to detect gases, chemicals, biological agents, electric fields, light, heat, or other targets. The term "nanobiosensors" implies use of nanosensors for detection of chemical or biological materials. Nanomaterials are exquisitely sensitive chemical and biological sensors. Since their surface properties are easily modified, nanowires can be decorated with virtually any potential chemical or biological molecular recognition unit, making the wires themselves independent of the analyte. The nanomaterials transduce the chemical binding event on their surface into a change in conductance of the nanowire in an extremely sensitive, real time and quantitative fashion. Boron-doped silicon nanowires (SiNWs) have been used to create highly sensitive, real-time electrically based sensors for biological and chemical species. Biotin-modified SiNWs were used to detect streptavidin down to at least a picomolar concentration range. The small size and capability of these semiconductor nanowires for sensitive, label-free, real-time detection of a wide range of chemical and biological species could be exploited in array-based screening and in vivo diagnostics.

The sensors can be electronically gated to respond to the binding of a single molecule. Prototype sensors have demonstrated detection of nucleic acids, proteins and ions. These sensors can operate in the liquid or gas phase, opening up an enormous variety of downstream applications. The detection schemes use inexpensive low voltage measurement schemes and detect binding events directly so there is no need for costly, complicated and time-consuming labeling chemistries such as fluorescent dyes or the use of bulky and expensive optical detection systems. As a result, these sensors are inexpensive to manufacture and portable. It may even be possible to develop implantable detection and monitoring devices based on these detectors.

Some of the technologies that can be incorporated in biosensing are already covered in earlier sections. An example is nanopore technology, which can form the basis of nanosensors. Some of the biosensor devices are described in the following sections.

Carbon nanotube biosensors

Over the years, researchers have sought to tailor carbon nanotubes to detect chemicals ranging from small gas molecules to large biomolecules. The tubes' small size and unique electronic properties make them especially adept at detecting minute changes in the environment. A new type of optical nanosensor uses single-walled carbon nanotubes that modulate their emission in response to the adsorption of specific biomolecules (Barone et al 2005). It has two distinct mechanisms of signal transduction – fluorescence quenching and charge transfer. The nanotube-based chemical sensors developed so far generate an electric signal in the presence of a particular molecule. The basic design is widely applicable for such analytical tasks as detecting genes and proteins associated with diseases.

To test the feasibility of implanting the sensors in the body, oxidase- and ferricyanide-coated nanotubes were placed inside a sealed glass tube a centimeter long and 200 microns thick. The tube is riddled with pores large enough to let glucose enter but small enough to keep the nanotubes inside. The tube was then implanted in a sample of human skin and the sensor could be excited with infrared light and detect its fluorescence.

Ion Channel Switch biosensor technology

The Ion Channel Switch (ICS™), developed by Ambri Ltd, is a novel biosensor technology based upon a synthetic self assembling membrane. The membrane acts like a biological switch and is capable of detecting the presence of specific molecules, and signaling their presence by triggering an electrical current (Cornell 2002). It has the ability to detect a change in ion flow upon binding with the target molecule resulting in a rapid result currently unachievable using existing technologies. The Ambri ICS™ biosensor is one of the first true nanobiosensor devices and is the basis of SensiDx™ System that has been designed for POC testing in critical care environments in hospitals. By delivering precise, quantitative test results in an immediate timeframe, the SensiDx™ System may assist in reducing the time of emergency diagnoses down from hours to minutes. This has a positive impact on both clinical decision-making and treatment costs.

Electronic nanobiosensors

The Biodetect™ system (Integrated Nano-Technologies) works by electronically detecting the binding of a target DNA molecule to sensors on a microchip. The target molecules form a bridge between two electrically separated wires. In order to create a strong clear signal, the bound target molecules are chemically developed to form conductive DNA wires. These DNA wires "turn on" a sensor much like an on/off switch. Each chip contains multiple sensors, which can be independently addressed with capture probes for different target DNA molecules from the same or different organisms. Each sensor has hundreds of interdigitated wires that are electrically separated from its neighbors. A proprietary DNA Lithography™ process is used to attach capture probes to each of the sensors on the chip. These chips now have billions of capture probes per sensor, which greatly improves sensitivity. To form detectable DNA wires, target DNA molecules first must form a DNA bridge spanning the gap between the sensor wires. DNA bridge formation has been observed by fluorescent imaging techniques. The final step in the detection process is to metalize the DNA bridge to form a DNA wire. Various metalization chemistries have been developed, which enable metalization of the DNA bridges with very low levels of background deposition. After metalization, bridges can be readily detected by measuring the resistance or other electrical properties of the sensor. DNA wires can be seen using electron microscopy.

This portable system is used for rapid detection of microorganisms. This technology will also form the basis of site-specific drug delivery and high-resolution image arrays using nano-scale electronic components.

Quartz nanobalance biosensor

Single-strand DNA-containing thin films are deposited onto quartz oscillators to construct a device capable of sensing the presence of the complementary DNA sequences, which hybridize with the immobilized ones. DNA, once complexed with aliphatic amines, appears as a monolayer in a single-stranded form by X-ray small angle scattering. A quartz nanobalance is then utilized to monitor mass increment related to specific hybridization with a complementary DNA probe. The crystal quartz nanobalance, capable of high sensitivity, indeed appears capable of obtaining a prototype of a device capable of sensing the occurrence of particular genes or sequences in the sample under investigation.

Viral nanosensor

Virus particles are essentially biological nanoparticles. Herpes simplex virus (HSV) and adenovirus can be used to trigger the assembly of magnetic nanobeads as nanosensors for clinically relevant viruses (Perez et al 2003). The nanobeads have a supramagnetic iron oxide core coated with dextran. Protein G is attached as a binding partner for antivirus antibodies. By conjugating anti-HSV antibodies directly to nanobeads using a bifunctional linker to avoid non-specific interactions between medium components and protein G and using a magnetic field, it is possible to detect as few as 5 viral particles in a 10mL serum sample. This system is more sensitive than ELISA-based methods and is an improvement over PCR-based detection because it is cheaper, faster and has fewer artifacts.

PEBBLE nanosensors

PEBBLE (Probes Encapsulated by Biologically Localized Embedding) nanosensors consist of sensor molecules entrapped in a chemically inert matrix by a microemulsion polymerization process that produces spherical sensors in the size range of 20 to 200 nm (Sumner et al 2002). These sensors are capable of real-time inter- and intra-cellular imaging of ions and molecules and are insensitive to interference from proteins. PEBBLE can also be used for early detection of cancer. PEBBLE nanosensors also show very good reversibility and stability to leaching and photobleaching, as well as very short response times and no perturbation by proteins. In human plasma they demonstrate a robust oxygen sensing capability, little affected by light scattering and autofluorescence (Cao et al 2004).

Nanosensors for glucose monitoring

One of the main reasons for developing in vivo glucose sensors is the detection of hypoglycemia in people with insulin dependent (type 1) diabetes. It is possible to engineer fluorescent micro/nanoscale devices for glucose sensing. Deployment of micro/nanoparticles in the dermis may allow transdermal monitoring of glucose changes in interstitial fluid. Using electrostatic self-assembly, an example of nanotechnology for fabrication, two types of sensors are being studied (McShane 2002): (1) solid nanoparticles coated with fluorescent enzyme-containing thin films and (2) hollow micro/nanocapsules containing fluorescent indicators and enzymes or glucose-binding proteins. Nanoengineering of the coated colloids and microcapsules allows precision control over optical, mechanical, and catalytic properties to achieve sensitive response using a combination of polymers, fluorescent indicators, and glucose-specific proteins. Challenges to in vivo use include understanding of material toxicity and failure modes, and determining methods to overcome fouling, protein inactivation, and material degradation. Non-invasive glucose sensing will maximize acceptance by patients and overcome biocompatibility problems of implants. Near infrared spectroscopy has been most investigated but the precision needs to be improved for eventual clinical application.

The nanotube-based optical biosensor could free people with diabetes from the daily pinprick tests now required for monitoring blood sugar concentrations. Carbon nanotubes are coated with glucose oxidase, an enzyme that breaks down glucose molecules. Then ferricyanide, an electron-hungry molecule, is sprinkled, onto the nanotubes' surfaces. Ferricyanide draws electrons from the nanotubes, quenching their capacity to glow when excited by infrared light. When glucose is present, it reacts with the oxidase, producing hydrogen peroxide. In turn, the hydrogen peroxide reacts with ferricyanide in a way that reduces that molecule's hunger for electrons. The higher the glucose level, the greater is the nanotube's infrared fluorescence.

A technique has been reported for micromechanical detection of biologically relevant glucose concentrations by immobilization of glucose oxidase (GOx) onto a microcantilever surface (Pei et al 2004). The enzyme-functionalized microcantilever undergoes bending due to a change in surface stress induced by the reaction between glucose in solution and the GOx immobilized on the cantilever surface.

Use of nanotube electronic biosensor in proteomics

A single-walled carbon nanotubes as a platform has been used for investigating surface-protein and protein-protein binding and developing highly specific electronic biomolecule detectors (Chen et al 2003). Nonspecific binding on nanotubes, a phenomenon found with a wide range of proteins, is overcome by immobilization of polyethylene oxide chains. A general approach is then advanced to enable the selective recognition and binding of target proteins by conjugation of their specific receptors to polyethylene oxide-functionalized nanotubes. These arrays are attractive because no labeling is required and all aspects of the assay can be carried out in solution phase. This scheme, combined with the sensitivity of nanotube electronic devices, enables highly specific electronic sensors for detecting clinically important biomolecules such as antibodies associated with human autoimmune diseases. These arrays are attractive because no labeling is required and all aspects of the assay can be carried out in solution phase. Interfacing novel nanomaterials with biological systems could therefore lead to important applications in disease diagnosis, proteomics, and nanobiotechnology in general.

Microneedle-mounted biosensor

NanoSense (NanoPass Technologies Ltd) is a MicroPyramid™ chip that is integrated with biosensors for nanoliter scale ion diagnostics for congestive heart failure and renal failure. This technology will be integrated with microneedles to provide reliable, inexpensive and simple to operate transdermal device for ion diagnoses, in point-of-care settings. This work is conducted in collaboration with MESA (Micro Electronics, Materials Engineering, Sensors and Actuators) Laboratories at the University of Twente, the Netherlands (http://www.mesaplus.utwente.nl/)

Optical biosensors

Many biosensors that are currently marketed rely on the optical properties of lasers to monitor and quantify interactions of biomolecules that occur on specially derived surfaces or biochips. An integrated biosensor, based on phototransistor integrated circuits, has been developed for use in medical detection, DNA diagnostics, and gene mapping. The biochip device has sensors, amplifiers, discriminators, and logic circuitry on board. Integration of light-emitting diodes into the device is also possible. Measurements of fluorescent-labeled DNA probe microarrays and hybridization experiments with a sequence-specific DNA probe for HIV-1 on nitrocellulose substrates illustrate the usefulness and potential of this DNA biochip. A number of variations of optical biosensors offer distinct methods of sample application and detection in addition to different types of sensor surface. Surface plasmon resonance technology is the best-known example of this technology.

Novel optical mRNA biosensor

Nanoscale Science section of the National Center of Competence in Research (Basel, Switzerland) has developed a novel optical mRNA biosensor for application in pathology. The scheme of this biosensor is shown in Figure 5-2. Molecular beacons that are highly sequence specific are used as molecular switches. This biosensor detects single molecules in fluids and can be used to search for molecular markers to predict the prognosis of disease.

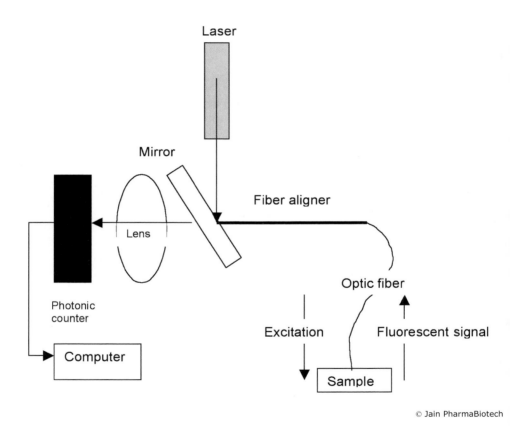

Figure 5-2: Scheme of a novel optical mRNA biosensor

Surface plasmon resonance technology

Surface Plasmon Resonance (SPR) is an optical-electrical phenomenon involving the interaction of light with the electrons of a metal. The optical-electronic basis of SPR is the transfer of the energy carried by photons of light to a group of electrons (a plasmon) at the surface of a metal. In Biacore systems (Figure 5-3), SPR arises when light is reflected under certain conditions from a conducting film at the interface between two media of different refractive index. The media are the sample and the glass of the sensor chip, and the conducting film is a thin layer of gold on the chip surface. SPR causes a reduction in the intensity of reflected light at a specific angle of reflection (the SPR angle). When molecules in the sample bind to the sensor surface, the concentration and therefore the refractive index at the surface changes and an SPR response is detected. Plotting the response against time during the course of an interaction provides a quantitative measure of the progress of the interaction. This plot is called a sensorgram.

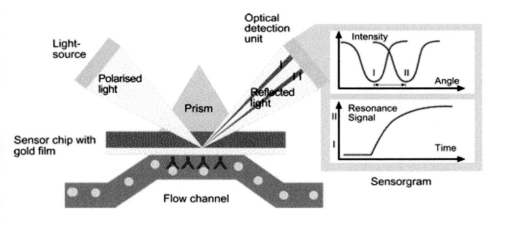

Figure 5-3: Surface plasmon resonance (SPR) technology

HTS Biosystems and Applied Biosystems Group are now co-developing a next-generation microarray-based SPR system that is designed to help researchers profile and characterize biomolecular interactions in a parallel format. Applied Biosystems has introduced SPR in its 8500 Affinity Chip Analyzer. This instrument cannot match Biacore's variety of chip surface chemistries - Biacore offers nine different surfaces to Applied Biosystems' three - the new system targets the drug-discovery market with its high-throughput format. The key strength of the system is that it can measure binding to all the different ligands under exactly the same conditions. The 8500 Affinity Chip Analyzer can simultaneously examine up to 400 binding interactions on a single chip during a two-hour run and can measure binding constants in the micromolar to picomolar range; the minimum analyte size for kinetic measurements is 8 kD.

Miniature optical sensors that specifically identify low concentrations of environmental and biological substances are in high demand. Currently, there is no optical sensor that provides identification of the aforementioned species without amplification techniques at naturally occurring concentrations. Triangular silver nanoparticles have remarkable optical properties and their enhanced sensitivity to their nanoenvironment has been used to develop a new class of optical sensors using localized SPR spectroscopy (Haes and Duyne 2004).

Nanoshell biosensors

Nanoshells can enhance chemical sensing by as much as 10 billion times. That makes them about 10,000 times more effective at Raman scattering than traditional methods. When molecules and materials scatter light, a small fraction of the light interacts in such a way that it allows scientists to determine their detailed chemical makeup. This property, known as Raman scattering, is used by medical researchers, drug designers, chemists and other scientists to determine what materials are made of. An enormous limitation in the use of Raman scattering has been its extremely weak sensitivity. Nanoshells can provide large, clean, reproducible enhancements of this effect, opening the door for new, and all optical sensing applications. Scientists at the Rice University's Laboratory of Nanophotonics have found that nanoshells are extremely effective at magnifying the Raman signature of molecules, each individual nanoshell acting as an independent Raman enhancer. That creates an opportunity to design all-optical nanoscale sensors – essentially new molecular-level diagnostic instruments – that could detect as little as a few molecules of a target substance, which could be anything from a drug molecule or a key disease protein to a deadly chemical agent.

The metal cover of the nanoshell captures passing light and focuses it, a property that directly leads to the enormous Raman enhancements observed. Furthermore, nanoshells can be tuned to interact with specific wavelengths of light by varying the thickness of their shells. This tunability allows for the Raman enhancements to be optimized for specific wavelengths of light. The finding that individual nanoshells can vastly enhance the Raman effect opens the door for biosensor designs that use a single nanoshell, something that could prove useful for engineers who are trying to probe the chemical processes within small structures such as individual cells, or for the detection of very small amounts of a material, like a few molecules of a deadly biological or chemical agent. Nanoshells are already being developed for applications including cancer diagnosis, cancer therapy, diagnosis and testing for proteins associated with Alzheimer's disease, drug delivery and rapid whole-blood immunoassay.

Laser nanosensors

In a laser nanosensor, laser light is launched into the fiber, and the resulting evanescent field at the tip of the fiber is used to excite target molecules bound to the antibody molecules. A photometric detection system is used to detect the optical signal (e.g., fluorescence) originating from the analyte molecules or from the analyte-bioreceptor reaction (Vo-Dinh 2005). Laser nanosensors can be used for in vivo analysis of proteins and biomarkers in individual living cells.

Lipoparticles biosensors

Lipoparticles (Integral Molecular Inc) provide a means for solubilizing integral membrane proteins that would lose their structure if extracted away from the lipid membrane. The methods for using Lipoparticles range from traditional fluorescent detection technologies to emerging biosensor technologies. Lipoparticles are being used as membrane-delineated molecular probes, incorporating user-defined membrane-anchored proteins, soluble molecules, or enzymes for target interaction and optical signal emission. Arrays of Lipoparticles containing membrane proteins are being used to accelerate and simplify the processes of pathogen identification and pathogen-receptor pairing. Applications for membrane protein arrays include biodefense, diagnostics, drug discovery, and proteomics. A scheme of biosensors based on Lipoparticle is shown in Figure 5-4. The optimal detection system can be used depending on the target protein and the goal of the assay.

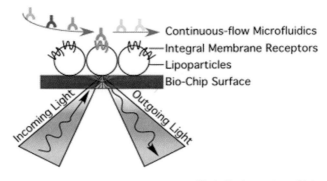

Illustration by courtesy of Integral Molecular Inc

Figure 5-4: Lipoparticle biosensors

Nanowire biosensors

When biological molecules bind to their receptors on the nanowire, they usually alter the current moving through the sensor and signal the presence of substance of interest. This direct detection dispenses with the time-consuming labeling chemistry and speeds up the detection process considerably. Nanowire biosensors are used for the detection of proteins, viruses or DNA in a highly sensitive manner. They can be devised to test for a complex of proteins associated with a particular cancer and used for diagnosis as well as monitoring the progress of treatment.

Nanowire biosensors for detection of single viruses

Rapid, selective, and sensitive detection of viruses is crucial for implementing an effective response to viral infection, such as through medication or quarantine. Established methods for viral analysis include plaque assays, immunological assays, transmission electron microscopy, and PCR-based testing of viral nucleic acids. These methods have not achieved rapid detection at a single virus level and often require a relatively high level of sample manipulation that is inconvenient for infectious materials.

Direct, real-time electrical detection of single virus particles with high selectivity has been reported by using nanowire field effect transistors (Patolsky et al 2004). Measurements made with nanowire arrays modified with antibodies for influenza A showed discrete conductance changes characteristic of binding and unbinding in the presence of influenza A but not paramyxovirus or adenovirus.

Simultaneous electrical and optical measurements using fluorescently labeled influenza A were used to demonstrate conclusively that the conductance changes correspond to binding/unbinding of single viruses at the surface of nanowire devices. pH-dependent studies further show that the detection mechanism is caused by a field effect, and that the nanowire devices can be used to determine rapidly isoelectric points and variations in receptor-virus binding kinetics for different conditions. Larger arrays of reproducible nanowire devices might simultaneously screen for the presence of 100 or more different viruses. Finally, studies of nanowire devices modified with antibodies specific for either influenza or adenovirus show that multiple viruses can be selectively detected in parallel. The possibility of large-scale integration of these nanowire devices suggests potential for simultaneous detection of a large number of distinct viral threats at the single virus level.

Nanowires for detection of genetic disorders

The surfaces of the silicon nanowire devices have been modified with peptide nucleic acid (PNA) receptors designed to recognize wild type versus the F508 mutation site in the cystic fibrosis transmembrane receptor gene (Hahm and Lieber 2004). Conductance measurements made while sequentially introducing wild type or mutant DNA samples exhibit a time-dependent conductance increase consistent with the PNA-DNA hybridization and enabled identification of fully complementary versus mismatched DNA samples. Concentration-dependent measurements show that detection can be carried out to at least the tens of femtomolar range. It provides more rapid results than current methods of DNA detection. This nanowire-based approach represents a step forward for direct, label-free DNA detection with extreme sensitivity and good selectivity, and could provide a pathway to integrated, high-throughput, multiplexed DNA detection for genetic screening.

Wireless nanosensors

Wireless biosensors are increasingly seen as a desirable treatment for a range of chronic conditions including diabetes, cardiac conditions and asthma. An intelligent, ultra-low power sensor (Bio-Nano Sensium Technologies) incorporates wireless communication to create bionanosensors that can be implanted within the body to diagnose and treat a wide variety of medical conditions. The development effort will focus on the information and communication technology systems necessary for these sensors to interact with their surrounding environment. The Bio-Nano Sensium will be based on industry-standard Complementary Metal Oxide Semiconductor technology so that not only will it have superior functional features to other devices but also be capable of low-cost production. A limited beta test program of this wireless biosensor system is available for evaluation.

Future issues in the development of nanobiosensors

- New biosensors and biosensor arrays are being developed using new materials, nanomaterials and microfabricated materials including new methods of patterning. Biosensor components will use nanofabrication technologies. Use of nanotubes, Buckminsterfullerenes (buckyballs), silica and its derivatives can produce nanosized devices. Some of the challenges will be:

- Development of real-time non-invasive technologies that can be applied to detection and quantitation of biological fluids without the need for multiple calibrations using clinical samples.

- Development of biosensors utilizing new technologies that offer improved sensitivity for detection with high specificity at the molecular level

- Development of biosensor arrays that can successfully detect, quantify and quickly identify individual components of mixed gases and liquid in an industrial environment

It would be desirable to develop multiple integrated biosensor systems that utilize doped oxides, polymers, enzymes or other components to give the system the required specificity. A system with all the sensor components, software, plumbing, reagents and sample processing are an example of an integrated sensor. There is also a need for reliable fluid handling systems for "dirty" fluids and for relatively small quantities of fluids (nanoliter to attoliter quantities). These should be low cost, disposable, reliable and easy to use as part of an integrated sensor system. Sensing in picoliter to attoliter volumes might create new problems in development of microreactors for sensing and novel phenomenon in very small channels.

6. PHARMACEUTICAL APPLICATIONS OF NANODIAGNOSTICS

Abstract

As nanobiotechnology is applied in molecular diagnostics, it will also have an impact on the pharmaceutical applications. One example is detection of biomarkers, which have diagnostic value as well as usefulness for drug discovery. SNP genotyping, based on nanobiotechnology, can be used in the drug development process. Other areas of application of nanodiagnostics in relation to pharmaceuticals include gene expression profiling and proteomics. Nanoparticles have also been used for drug discovery. Integration of diagnostics and therapeutics is important for the development of personalized medicine and this integration is done more effectively at nanoscale. This process may start at the early stage of drug development process.

Introduction

Molecular diagnostics has been applied in a number of areas besides the diagnosis of infections, genetic disorders and cancer. This includes the use of diagnostic genotyping, which is currently used to explore prediction of disease predisposition and identification of genetic markers for drug efficacy and toxicity. This is an extension of human genotyping. Most of the work in this area is still done in research laboratories in the academic institutions as well as biotechnology and pharmaceutical companies. Pharmaceutical companies have taken the initiative in this direction and also use molecular diagnostic technologies in the drug development process.

As nanobiotechnology is applied in molecular diagnostics, it will also have an impact on the pharmaceutical applications. An important use of molecular diagnostic technologies is detection of biomarkers, which have diagnostic value as well as usefulness for drug discovery.

Detection of biomarkers by nanotechnologies

The simplest definition of a biological marker (biomarker) is a molecule that indicates an alteration in physiology from normal. From a practical point of view, the biomarker would specifically and sensitively reflect a disease state and could be used for diagnosis as well as for disease monitoring during and following therapy. Currently available molecular diagnostic technologies have been used to detect biomarkers of various diseases such as cancer, metabolic disorders, infections and diseases of the central nervous system. Nanotechnology has further refined the detection of biomarkers. Some of the newly discovered biomarkers also form the basis of innovative molecular diagnostic tests.

Single molecule labeling

Nanomolecular probes

Research into tailoring the optical properties, surface chemistry and biocompatibility of metallic and semiconductor nanoparticles is fulfilling the promise of chemical nanostructures as customizable substitutes for organic molecular probes (Taton 2002). Chemists have reported synthetic routes towards semiconductor 'quantum dots' for fluorescent tagging, metal nanoparticles with extraordinarily high extinction coefficients for labeling in colorimetric and surface plasmon resonance assays and elongated 'nanorods' for measuring anisotropy. Nanoparticles are also providing alternatives to organic and organometallic probes for other (non-optical) biological applications, such as paramagnetic particles for magnetic resonance contrast imaging and metal particles for thermal probing of specific biomolecular interactions. The chemical synthesis of most of these nanostructures is typically achieved with just one reaction, involving a chemical transformation of a precursor source of inorganic material followed by a nanocrystallization process in the same vessel. Fine control over synthetic conditions is responsible for the reproducible range of novel properties these materials exhibit. As a result, nanostructured biological probes are easier to make and might eventually be less expensive to buy than organic dyes. In addition, the specific photochemical reactions that cause organic probes to photobleach or crosslink nonspecifically with biological samples are far less common for inorganic nanostructures. Admittedly, there are still limitations to using nanostructures as biological probes. Nanoparticles are significantly larger than molecular dyes and a bound nanostructure might sterically block access to the active sites of a biomolecule or affect its diffusion. In addition, the bioconjugation chemistry of some nanomaterials is still not fully refined. Nevertheless, the control that synthetic chemists have demonstrated over the structure and properties of nanoparticle materials is impressive, and naturally points towards their biological applications.

Optical trapping and single-molecule fluorescence

Two of the mainstay techniques in single-molecule research are optical trapping and single-molecule fluorescence. Previous attempts to combine these techniques in a single experiment and on a single macromolecule of interest have met with little success, because the light intensity within an optical trap is more than ten orders of magnitude greater than the light emitted by a single fluorophore. Instead, the two techniques have been employed sequentially, or spatially separated by distances of several micrometers within the sample, imposing experimental restrictions that limit the utility of the combined method. An instrument capable of true, simultaneous, spatially coincident optical trapping and single-molecule fluorescence has been developed (Lang et al 2003). This opens the door to many types of experiment that employ optical traps to supply controlled external loads while fluorescent molecules report concurrent information about macromolecular structure. The combination of these two biophysical techniques in a single assay offers a powerful tool for studying molecular systems by allowing direct correlations to be made between nanoscale structural changes.

Single molecule detection

Single-molecule detection of DNA hybridization

Nanometer-scale conformational changes of a single 10- to 30-nm-long DNA oligonucleotide can be detected through a micromechanical technique in which the quantity monitored is the displacement of a micrometer-size bead tethered to a surface by the probe molecule undergoing the conformational change (Singh-Zocchi et al 2003). This technique allows probing of conformational changes within distances beyond the range of fluorescence resonance energy transfer. The method has been applied to detect single hybridization events of label-free target oligomers. Hybridization of the target is detected through the conformational change of the probe. Potential applications are as a platform for sensitive DNA arrays. A further advantage of the method is that it delivers a quantitative measurement of probe shortening, rather than detecting only the presence of the target. Hybridization of partial homologues could be discriminated on this basis. Further steps will include moving from detection alone to measuring the amount of target, which will involve collecting the signal from many smaller beads. Other aspects to be improved include: more stable (covalent) attachment of the probe oligomers to the surfaces, better surface chemistry to minimize nonspecific sticking of the beads, perhaps the possibility of controlling bead–slide interactions, and hybridization rates through an electric field.

Single DNA molecules labeled with nanoparticles can be detected by blockades of ionic current as they are translocated through a nanopipette tip formed by a pulled glass capillary (Karhanek et al 2005). The nanopipette detection technique can provide not only tools for detection and identification of single DNA and protein molecules but also deeper insight and understanding of stochastic interactions of various biomolecules with their environment.

Application of AFM for biomolecular imaging

AFM has become a well-established technique for imaging single biomolecules under physiological conditions. The exceptionally high spatial resolution and signal-to-noise ratio of the AFM enables the substructure of individual molecules to be observed. In contrast to other methods, specimens prepared for AFM remain in a plastic state, which enables direct observation of the dynamic molecular response, creating unique opportunities for studying the structure–function relationships of proteins and their functionally relevant assemblies.

The combination of single-molecule imaging with other techniques to monitor topographical, biochemical and physical parameters simultaneously is a powerful, interesting and unique application of AFM. This correlation of biochemical and physical information can provide new insights into fundamental biological processes. Several different approaches for obtaining multiple parameters during AFM imaging have been developed, including AFM in combination with optical microscopy, patch clamp electrophysiology and ion-conductance pipettes. Used as a sensor, the AFM tip can also probe the charges of biological surfaces immersed in a buffer solution. So far, such approaches have successfully characterized protein interactions but in the future they could be applied to imaging and detecting multiple parameters on a single molecule simultaneously.

AFM has been used to study and characterize gene complexes composed of plasmid DNA and cationic lipids. Surface morphology of spherical complexes with diameters of approximately 200-300 nm have been examined (Oberle et al 2003). However, AFM technique does not enable any conclusions to be drawn regarding the architecture of the inner core of the lipoplex as only the morphology of the surface structures can be obtained reliably.

One of the critical limitations of AFM is its inability to recognize the specific chemical composition of a molecule. AFM uses a tiny, highly sensitive probe that, when pulled across the surface of a sample, maps its topography down to the nanometer scale. Until recently, it could not identify exactly what the proteins on its map as all proteins look the same in an AFM image. Scientists at the Arizona State University (Tempe, Arizona) found a solution to this limitation by using an even tinier polymer thread that attached antibodies designed to bind to individual proteins to the tip of the AFM probe (Stroh et al 2004). When the antibody binds to the target protein, it creates a variance in the microscope's reading. This is a technique for identifying any antigen in a complex sample on the nanometer scale and has applicability that goes far beyond sorting out AFM images. It could be used to read arrays on the nanometer scale to enable mapping of the entire interaction potential landscape between a receptor and a ligand.

Future insights into biomolecular processes by AFM

AFM has become a well-established technique for imaging individual macromolecules at a spatial resolution of <1 nm. The next step will be to establish new AFM methods to investigate structure-function relationships among the variety of molecular machines. Such results will provide insights into how such machines work at the molecular level, and drive the understanding of common principles that govern them. The next challenge will be to study the behavior of individual molecular machines in heterogeneous assemblies, and to understand how different machines form small functional entities. Here, again, AFM promises to be an important tool as it enables individual molecules to be imaged at sufficient resolution for their behavior within macromolecular complexes to be characterized.

Applications of biomolecular computing in life sciences

An autonomous biomolecular computer, at least in vitro, can logically analyze the levels of mRNA species, and in response produces a molecule capable of affecting levels of gene expression (Benenson et al 2004). This approach might be applied in vivo to biochemical sensing, genetic engineering and even medical diagnosis and treatment. As a proof of principle, the researchers programmed the computer to identify and analyze mRNA of disease-related genes associated with models of small-cell lung cancer and prostate cancer, and to produce a single-stranded DNA molecule modeled after an anticancer drug. These preliminary experiments were performed under tightly controlled, test-tube conditions. To have therapeutic value, the computers must be installed inside cells and protected from cellular defense mechanisms once they get there.

Role of nanodiagnostic technologies in drug discovery

Molecular diagnostic technologies are used for drug discovery as shown in Table 6-1. All of these can be refined by the application of nanotechnology.

Table 6-1: Molecular diagnostic technologies for drug discovery

Genotyping
Mutation detection
Identification of single nucleotide polymorphisms (SNPs)
High-throughput DNA sequencing
Gene expression profiles
Biochips/ microarrays/ microfluidics
Molecular imaging of gene expression
Proteomic technologies
Mass spectrometry for target identification
Protein-protein interactions analyses
Protein chip
Biosensors for detection of small molecule-protein interactions

The new challenges in the identification of therapeutic targets require efficient and cost-effective tools. Label-free detection systems use proteins or ligands coupled to materials the physical properties of which are measurably modified following specific interactions. Among the label-free systems currently available, the use of metal nanoparticles offers enhanced throughput and flexibility for real-time monitoring of biomolecular recognition at a reasonable cost. Nanodiagnostic technologies have been applied for drug discovery and development. Some technologies will accelerate target identification whereas others will evolve into therapeutics.

Current drug discovery process needs improvement in several areas. Although many targets are being discovered through genomics and proteomics, the efficiency of screening and validation processes need to be increased. Through further miniaturization, nanotechnology will improve the ability to fabricate massive arrays in small spaces using microfluidics and the time efficiency. This would enable direct reading of the signals from microfluidic circuits in a manner similar to a microelectronics circuit where one does not require massive instrumentation. This would increase the ability to do high-throughput drug screening.

The use of various nanotechnologies for drug discovery has been reviewed elsewhere (Jain 2005e). Nanocrystals (quantum dots) and other nanoparticles (gold colloids, magnetic nanoparticles, nanobarcodes, nanobodies, dendrimers, fullerenes and nanoshells) have received a considerable attention recently with their unique properties for potential use in drug discovery. This section will examine the usefulness and limitations of some of these technologies for drug discovery.

Use of quantum dots for drug discovery

The use of quantum dots (QDs) for drug discovery has been explored extensively. Both advantages and drawbacks have been investigated (Ozkan 2004).

Advantages of the use of QDs for drug discovery

- Enhanced optical properties as compared with organic dyes. QDs offer great imaging results that could not be achieved by organic dyes. They have narrow band emission together with large UV absorption spectra, which enables multiplexed imaging under a single light source.

- Multiple leads can be tested on cell culture simultaneously. Similarly, the absorption of several drug molecules can be studied simultaneously for a longer period of time.

- Using the surface functionalization properties of QDs, targeting capabilities can be added as well.

- Due to the inorganic nature of QDs, their interaction with their immediate environment at in vivo states can be minimal compared with their organic counterparts.

Drawbacks of the use of QDs for drug discovery

QDs have not been totally perfected and some of the drawbacks are:

- Size variation during the synthesis of single color dots is 2-4%. For applications such as capillary electrophoresis or gel electrophoresis, it could create false results.

- The number of functional groups attached to an organic dye is usually one and it can be controlled very precisely. However, in the case of QDs, the functional groups usually decorate the entire surface and thus cause multiple attachments of target molecules.

- The 'blinking' characteristics of QDs when they are excited with high-intensity light could be a limiting factor for fast scan systems such as flow cytometry.

- Under combined aqueous-UV excitation conditions, QDs demonstrate oxidation and release of cadmium ions into the environment. This is a definite concern for in vivo applications.

Quantum dot for imaging drug receptors in the brain

Single-molecule properties in living cells can be followed by using quantum dots (QDs). QDs have been used to track individual glycine receptors (GlyRs) and analyze their dynamics in the neuronal membrane of living cells for periods ranging from milliseconds to minutes (Dahan et al 2003). The glycine receptors are the main inhibitory neurotransmitter in the human spinal cord and brain stem. The entry of GlyRs into the synapse by diffusion was observed and further confirmed by electron microscopy imaging of QD-tagged receptors. Older imaging tools such as fluorescent dyes or polymer spheres are either too unstable or too large to effectively perform single-molecule tracking. QD conjugates, by contrast, produced photo resolutions up to eight times more detailed than the older imaging tools. The conjugates also proved to be "almost an order of magnitude" brighter than fluorescent dyes, and could be observed for as long as 40 minutes compared to about 5 seconds for the dyes. Length of observation time is critical to studying cellular processes, which change rapidly over a span of several minutes. Cellular receptors are a critical target studied by scientists who develop new drug candidates for diseases including neurological disorders such as epilepsy and depression. More detailed understanding of the behavior of these receptors can open up new treatment options.

Gold nanoparticles for drug discovery

Tracking drug molecules in cells

Gold nanoparticles have been used to demonstrate multiphoton absorption induced luminescence (MAIL), in which specific tissues or cells are fluorescently-labeled using special stains that enable them to be studied. Gold nanoparticles can emit light so strongly that it is readily possible to observe a single nanoparticle at laser intensities lower than those commonly used for MAIL sub-100-fs pulses of 790-nm light (Farrer et al 2005). Moreover, gold nanoparticles do not blink or burn out, even after hours of observation. These observations suggest that metal nanoparticles are a viable alternative to fluorophores or semiconductor nanoparticles for biological labeling and imaging. Other advantages of the technique are that the gold nanoparticles can be prepared easily, have very low toxicity, and can readily be attached to molecules of biological interest. In addition, the laser light used to visualize the particles is a wavelength that causes only minimal damage to most biological tissues. This technology could enable tracking of a single molecule of a drug in a cell or other biological samples.

SPR with colloidal gold particles

Conventional SPR is applied in specialized biosensing instruments. These instruments use expensive sensor chips of limited reuse capacity and require complex chemistry for ligand or protein immobilization. SPR has also been successfully applied with colloidal gold particles in buffered solution (Englebienne et al 2003a). This application offers many advantages over conventional SPR. The support is cheap, easily synthesized, and can be coated with various proteins or protein-ligand complexes by charge adsorption. With colloidal gold, the SPR phenomenon can be monitored in any UV-vis spectrophotometer. For high-throughput applications, the technology has been adapted in an automated clinical chemistry analyzer. Among the label-free systems currently available, the use of metal nanocolloids offers enhanced throughput and flexibility for real-time biomolecular recognition monitoring at a reasonable cost (Englebienne et al 2003).

Assays using magnetic nanoparticles

Several assays are used for screening drug targets. Magnetic nanoparticles are used in many biochemical assays as labels for concentration, manipulation and, more recently, detection. Typically one attaches the magnetic particles to the biochemical species of interest (target) using a chemically specific binding interaction. Once bound, the labels enable the manipulation of the target species through the application of magnetic forces. Spintronic sensors, specifically Giant Magnetoresistive and Spin Dependent Tunneling, sensors have been developed to detect and quantify labels in two main formats: flowing in a microfluidic channel, and immobilized labels on a chip surface (Smith et al 2004).

Lipoparticle biosensor for drug discovery

Interactions with integral membrane proteins have been particularly difficult to study because the receptors cannot be removed from the lipid membrane of a cell without disrupting the structure and function of the protein. Cell-based assays are the current standard for drug discovery against integral membrane proteins, but are limited in important ways. Biosensors are capable of addressing many of these limitations. Biosensors are currently being used in target identification, validation, assay development, lead optimization, and ADMET studies, but are best suited for soluble molecules. Lipoparticles (Integral Molecular Inc) are being using to effectively solubilize integral membrane proteins for use in biosensors and other microfluidic devices. A primary application of current biosensor technologies is the optimization of limited-scope drug libraries against specific targets. Paired with Integral's Lipoparticle technology, biosensors can be used to address some of the most complex biological problems facing the drug discovery industry, including cell-cell recognition, cell-adhesion, cell-signaling, lipid interactions, and protein-protein interactions.

Nanowire biosensors to analyze small molecule-protein interactions

Development of miniaturized devices that enable rapid and direct analysis of the specific binding of small molecules to proteins could be of substantial importance to the discovery of and screening for new drug molecules. Highly sensitive and label-free direct electrical detection of small-molecule inhibitors of ATP binding to Abl can be accomplished by using silicon nanowire field-effect transistor devices (Wang et al 2005). Abl, which is a protein tyrosine kinase whose constitutive activity is responsible for chronic myelogenous leukemia, was covalently linked to the surfaces of silicon nanowires within microfluidic channels to create active electrical devices. Concentration-dependent binding of ATP and concentration-dependent inhibition of ATP binding by the competitive small-molecule antagonist Gleevec were assessed by monitoring the nanowire conductance. In addition, concentration-dependent inhibition of ATP binding was examined for four additional small molecules, including reported and previously unreported inhibitors. These studies demonstrate that the silicon nanowire devices can readily and rapidly distinguish the affinities of distinct small-molecule inhibitors and, thus, could serve as a technology platform for drug discovery.

Role of AFM for study of biomolecular interactions for drug discovery

An approach called TREC (topography and recognition imaging) uses any of a number of different ligands such as antibodies, small organic molecules, and nucleotides bound to a carefully designed AFM tip-sensor which can, in a series of unbinding experiments, estimate affinity and structural data (Ebner et al 2005). If a ligand is attached to the end of an AFM probe, one can simulate various physiological conditions and look at the strength of the interaction between the ligand and receptor under a wide range of circumstances. By functionalizing the tip, one can use it to probe biological systems and identify particular chemical entities on the surface of a biological sample. This opens the door to more effective use of AFM in drug discovery.

AFM has been used to study the molecular-scale processes underlying the formation of the insoluble plaques associated with Alzheimer's disease (AD). As one of a class of neurological diseases caused by changes in a protein's physical state, called "conformational" diseases, it's particularly well suited for study with AFM. Extensive data suggest that the conversion of the Aβ peptide from soluble to insoluble forms is a key factor in the pathogenesis of AD. In recent years, AFM has provided useful insights into the physicochemical processes involving Aβ morphology. AFM was the key in identifying the nanostructures which are now recognized as different stages of Aβ aggregation in AD and has revealed other forms of aggregation, which are observable at earlier stages and evolve to associate into mature fibrils. AFM can now be used to explore factors that either inhibit or promote fibrillogenesis. Using of AFM enabled the comparison of two monoclonal antibodies being studied as potential treatments for AD to select the one that did a better job of inhibiting the formation of these protofibrils. M266.2, which binds to the central portion of the Aβ, completely inhibited the formation of protofibrils, while the other antibody, m3D6, slowed but did not totally stop their growth (Legleiter et al 2004). These results indicate that AFM can be not only reliably used to study the effect of different molecules on Aβ aggregation, but that it can provide additional information such as the role of epitope specificity of antibodies as potential inhibitors of fibril formation.

Role of nanodiagnostics in clinical trials

Biochip-based point-of-care diagnostics would be useful not only for selection of patients but also for evaluating the results of treatment. All these applications can be refined by use of nanotechnology. Molecular diagnostics play an important role in clinical trials, particularly where stratification is done on the basis of pharmacogenomics.

Role of nanodiagnostics in quality control of biopharmaceuticals

Detection of microbial contamination

Several technologies are used for the quality control of biopharmaceuticals. Adenosine triphosphate (ATP) bioluminescence and PCR-based assays provide rapid quality control analysis of cosmetic and pharmaceutical finished products and raw materials.

The ViriChip™ (Bioforce Nanoscience Inc) is a solid-phase method of virus and pathogen detection and identification that combines immunological recognition with ultra-sensitive detection using surface profiling by nanoarrays. This method will be used to assess the quality of vaccine formulations during production. Unlike other virus detection methods, which rely on amplification steps and signal enhancers, the ViriChip is able to directly detect and inspect virus particles.

DNA tagging for control and tracing of drug distribution channels

DNA tags are harmless and inexpensive, and it is difficult to detect or counterfeit the nucleotide sequence. Nanobarcode technology can be used to refine the process of tagging. This technique can be used for several purposes, including the following:

- Identifying abuse of prescription drugs such as diazepam and barbiturates

- Tracing the distribution and resale of prescription drugs

Safety and toxicity aspects of nanoparticles

Use of nanoparticles for in vitro diagnostics does not involve any safety issues. However, there are some safety concerns about the in vivo use of nanoparticles whether for diagnostics or therapeutic purposes. Some of these have to do with uncertain fate of nanoparticles in the human body.

Fate of nanoparticles in the human body

Smaller particles apparently circulate for much longer and in some cases can cross the blood-brain barrier to lodge in the brain. They can leak out of capillaries and get into the fluids between cells. So they can go to places in the body that an average inorganic mineral can not. Such effects may not be a concern in case of targeted delivery of nanoparticle-based therapy in cancer. The eventual decision to use nanoparticle-based therapy may depend on a risk-versus-benefit assessment.

Testing for toxicity of nanoparticles

A mouse spermatogonial stem cell line has been used as a model to assess nanotoxicity in the male germ line in vitro (Braydich-Stolle et al 2005). The effects of different types of nanoparticles on these cells were evaluated using light microscopy, cell proliferation and standard cytotoxicity assays. The results demonstrated a concentration-dependent toxicity for all types of particles tested, while the corresponding soluble salts had no significant effect. Ag nanoparticles were the most toxic while MoO_3 nanoparticles were the least toxic. These results suggest that this cell line provides a valuable model to assess the cytotoxicity of nanoparticles in the germ line in vitro.

Quantum dot toxicity

Cadmium selenide (CdSe) quantum dots are used as fluorescent labels. While cytotoxicity of bulk CdSe is well documented, CdSe QDs are generally cytocompatible, at least with some immortalized cell lines. Use of primary hepatocytes as a liver model has shown that CdSe-core QDs are acutely toxic under certain conditions (Derfus et al 2004). Although previous in vitro studies have not shown significant toxicity, the cell line used in these studies were not sensitive to heavy metals or the exposed to short-time QD labeling. The authors found that the cytotoxicity of QDs was modulated by processing parameters during

137

synthesis, exposure to ultraviolet light, and surface coatings. These data further suggest that cytotoxicity correlates with the liberation of free Cd^{2+} ions due to deterioration of the CdSe lattice. When appropriately coated, CdSe-core QDs can be rendered nontoxic and used to track cell migration and reorganization in vitro. These results provide information for design criteria for the use of QDs in vitro and especially in vivo, where deterioration over time may occur. Capping QDs with ZnO effectively prevented Cd^{2+} formation upon exposure to air but not to ultraviolet radiation. Investigations are in progress to test capping with other organic and inorganic materials.

Gold nanoparticle toxicity

Toxicity has been observed at high concentrations using gold nanoparticles. Studies using 2 nm core gold nanoparticles have shown that cationic particles are moderately toxic, whereas anionic particles are quite nontoxic (Goodman et al 2004). Concentration-dependent lysis mediated by initial electrostatic binding was observed in dye release studies using lipid vesicles, providing the probable mechanism for observed toxicity with the cationic particles.

Integration of nanodiagnostics and nanotherapeutics

Integration of diagnostics and therapeutics is important for the development of personalized medicine and this integration is done more effectively at nanoscale. This process may start at the early stage of drug development process. Pharmaceutical companies may market a package product containing both the diagnostic test and the therapeutic agent that is suitable for a certain genotype. A few such products are already in the market.

7. CLINICAL APPLICATIONS OF NANODIAGNOSTICS

Abstract

Applications of nanotechnologies in clinical diagnostics will have a tremendous impact on the practice of medicine. Biosensor systems based on nanotechnology could detect emerging disease in the body at a stage that may be curable. This is extremely important in management of infections and cancer. A number of devices based on nanotechnology are among those with potential applications in point-of-care (POC) testing. Use of nanoparticles as contrast agent for MRI will enable in vivo diangosis as an aid to patient management.

Introduction

Applications of nanotechnologies in clinical diagnostics have been reviewed recently (Jain 2005c). This will have a tremendous impact on the practice of medicine. Biosensor systems based on nanotechnology could detect emerging disease in the body at a stage that may be curable. This is extremely important in management of infections and cancer. Some of the body functions and responses to treatment will be monitored without cumbersome laboratory equipments. Some examples are a radiotransmitter small enough to put into a cell and acoustical devices to measure and record the noise a heart makes. Although applications of individual technologies are mentioned in Chapter 3, some important areas of clinical application will be identified here.

Nanotechnology for early detection of cancer

Nanobiotechnology offers a novel set of tools for detection of cancer. A workshop held at the National Institutes of Standards and Technology of USA in 2001 made the following recommendations (Srinivas et al 2002):

1. Nanotechnology can complement existing technologies and make significant contributions to cancer detection, prevention, diagnosis and treatment.

2. Nanotechnology would be extremely useful in the area of biomarker research and provide additional sensitivity in assays with relatively small sample volumes.

3. Specific nanotechnology applications that would impact on biomarker research are: (a) nanostructures such as biopores; (b) nanoprobes such as scanning tunnel microscopy; (c) nanosources such as laser-induced fluorescence; and (d) nanomaterials such as quantum dots.

QDs, coated with a polyacrylate cap and covalently linked to antibodies or to streptavidin, have been used for immunofluorescent labeling of breast cancer marker Her2 (Wu et al 2003). Labeling was highly specific, and was brighter and more stable than that of other fluorescent markers. Recent advances have led to QD bioconjugates that are highly luminescent and stable. These bioconjugates raise new possibilities for studying genes, proteins and drug targets in single cells, tissue specimens and even in living animals and enable visualization of cancer cells in living animals. Her2 and a method for detecting protein analytes has been developed that relies on magnetic microparticle probes with antibodies that specifically bind a target of interest (PSA in case of prostate cancer).

QDs can be combined with fluorescence microscopy to follow cells at high resolution in living animals. These offer considerable advantages over organic fluorophores for this purpose. QDs and emission spectrum scanning multiphoton microscopy have been used to develop a means to study extravasation in vivo (Voura et al 2004). Tumor cells labeled with QDs were intravenously injected into mice and followed as they extravasated into lung tissue. The behavior of QD-labeled tumor cells in vivo was indistinguishable from that of unlabeled cells. QDs and spectral imaging allowed the simultaneous identification of five different populations of cells using multiphoton laser excitation.

$\alpha v \beta 3$-targeted paramagnetic nanoparticles have been employed to noninvasively detect very small regions of angiogenesis associated with nascent melanoma tumors (Schmieder et al 2005). Each particle was filled with thousands of molecules of the metal that is used to enhance contrast in conventional MRI scans. The surface of each particle was decorated with a substance that attaches to newly forming blood vessels, which are present at tumor sites. The goal was to create a high density of the glowing particles at the site of tumor growth so they are easily visible. Molecular MRI results were corroborated by histology. This study lowers the limit previously reported for detecting sparse biomarkers with molecular MRI in vivo when the growths are still invisible to conventional MRI. Earlier detection can potentially increase the effectiveness of treatment. This is especially true with melanoma, which begins as a highly curable disorder, then progresses into an aggressive and deadly disease. A second benefit of the approach is that the same nanoparticles used to find the tumors could potentially deliver stronger doses of anticancer drugs directly to the tumor site with fewer side effects. Targeting the drugs to the tumor site in this way would also allow stronger doses without systemic toxicity than would be possible if the drug were injected or delivered in some other systemic way. The nanoparticles might also allow physicians to more readily assess the effectiveness of the treatment by comparing MRI scans before and after treatment. Other cancer types might be accessible to this approach as well, because all tumors recruit new blood vessels as they grow.

Gold nanoparticles conjugated to monoclonal anti-epidermal growth factor receptor (anti-EGFR) antibodies after incubation in cell cultures with malignant as well as nonmalignant epithelial cell lines. However, the anti-EGFR MAb-conjugated nanoparticles specifically and homogeneously bind to the surface of the cancer type cells with 600% greater affinity than to the noncancerous cells. This specific and homogeneous binding is found to give a relatively sharper SPR absorption band with a red shifted maximum compared to that observed when added to the noncancerous cells (El-Sayed et al 2005). The particles that worked the best were 35 nm in size. These results suggest that SPR scattering imaging or SPR absorption spectroscopy generated from antibody conjugated gold nanoparticles can be useful in molecular biosensor techniques for the diagnosis and investigation of oral epithelial living cancer cells in vivo and in vitro. Advantages of this technique are:

- It is not toxic to human cells. A similar technique using Quantum Dots uses semiconductor crystals to mark cancer cells, but the semiconductor material is potentially toxic to the cells and humans

- It does not require expensive high-powered microscopes or lasers to view the results. All it takes is a simple, inexpensive microscope and white light.

- The results are instantaneous. If a cancerous tissue is sprayed with gold nanoparticles containing the antibody, the results can be seen immediately. The scattering is so strong that a single particle can be detected.

Nanotechnology-based brain probes

Several brain probes and implants are used in neurosurgery. Examples are those for the management of epilepsy, movement disorders and pain. Many of these implants are still investigational. The ideal inert material for such implants has not yet been discovered. Silicon probes are commonly used for recording of electrical impulses and for brain stimulation. The brain generally regards these probes as a foreign material and encapsulates them with glial scar tissue, which prevents them from making good contact with the brain tissue.

An in vitro study was conducted to determine cytocompatibility properties of formulations containing carbon nanofibers pertinent to neural implant applications (McKenzie et al 2004). Substrates were prepared from four different types of carbon fibers, two with nanoscale diameters (less than or equal to 100 nm) and two with conventional diameters (greater than 100 nm). Within these two categories, both a high and a low surface energy fiber were investigated and tested. Astrocytes (glial scar tissue-forming cells) were seeded onto the substrates for adhesion, proliferation, and long-term function studies (such as total intracellular protein and alkaline phosphatase activity). Results provided the first evidence that astrocytes preferentially adhered and proliferated on carbon fibers that had the largest diameter and the lowest surface energy. Formulations containing carbon fibers in the nanometer regime limited astrocyte functions leading to decreased glial scar tissue formation. Positive interactions with neurons, and, at the same time, limited astrocyte functions leading to decreased gliotic scar tissue formation are essential for increased neuronal implant efficacy. Nanotubes, because of the interesting electronic properties and reduction in scar formation, hold great promise for replacing conventional silicon implants.

Electrical recording from spinal cord vascular capillary bed has been achieved demonstrating that the intravascular space may be utilized as a means to address brain activity with out violating the brain parenchyma. Working with platinum nanowires and using blood vessels as conduits to guide the wires, researchers have successfully detected the activity of individual neurons lying adjacent to the blood vessels (Llinas et al 2005). This can provide an understanding of the brain at the neuron-to-neuron interaction level with non-intrusive, biocompatible and biodegradable nanoprobes. This technique may one day enable monitoring of individual brain cells and perhaps provide new treatments for neurological diseases. Because the nanowires can deliver electrical impulses as well as receive them, the technique has potential as a treatment for Parkinson's disease (PD). It has already been shown that patients with PD can experience significant improvement from direct stimulation of the affected area of the brain. But the stimulation is currently carried out by inserting wires through the skull and into the brain, a process that can cause scarring of the brain tissue. By stimulating the brain with nanowires threaded through blood vessels, patients can receive benefits of the treatment without the damaging side effects. The challenge is to precisely guide the nanowire probes to a predetermined spot through the thousands of branches in the brain's vascular system. One solution is to replace the platinum nanowires with new conducting polymer nanowires. Not only do the polymers conduct electrical impulses, they change shape in response to electrical fields, which would allow the researchers to steer the nanowires through the brain's circulatory system. Polymer nanowires have the added benefit of being 20 to 30 times smaller than the platinum ones used in the reported laboratory experiments. They are biodegradable and therefore suitable for short-term brain implants.

Monitoring cardiovascular disease

Cardiac monitoring in sleep apnea

Because sleep apnea is a cause of irregular heartbeat, hypertension, heart attack, and stroke, it is important that patients be diagnosed and treated before these highly deleterious sequelae occur. For patients suspected of experiencing sleep apnea, in vivo sensors could constantly monitor blood concentrations of oxygen and cardiac function to detect problems during sleep. In addition, cardio-specific antibodies tagged with nanoparticles may allow doctors to visualize heart movement while a patient experiences sleep apnea to determine both short- and long-term effects of apnea on cardiac function.

Monitoring of disorders of blood coagulation

Patients would benefit greatly from nanotechnological devices that could monitor the body for the onset of thrombotic or hemorrhagic events. Multifunctional devices could detect events, transmit real-time biologic data externally, and deliver anticoagulants or clotting factors to buy critical time. Another likely role for nanoprobes is in cell tracking; quantum dots and superparamagnetic particles could be valuable for tracking hematopoietic and other stem cells to determine efficiency of cell delivery and survival.

Another benefit of nanotechnology in hemophilia is viral removal filtration system, nanofiltration, in the manufacture of plasma-derived coagulation factor concentrates and other biopharmaceutical products from human blood origin. Nanofiltration of plasma products has already been carried out since the early 1990s to improve margin of viral safety, as a complement to the viral reduction treatments, such as solvent-detergent and heat treatments, already applied for the inactivation of human immunodeficiency virus, hepatitis B and hepatitis C virus. The main reason for the introduction of nanofiltration was the need to improve product safety against non-enveloped viruses and to provide a possible safeguard against new infectious agents potentially entering the human plasma pool. Nanofiltration has gained quick acceptance as it is a relatively simple manufacturing step that consists in filtering protein solution through membranes of a very small pore size (typically 15-40 nm) under conditions that retain viruses by a mechanism largely based on size exclusion. Recent large-scale experience throughout the world has now established that nanofiltration is a robust and reliable viral reduction technique that can be applied to essentially all plasma products. Many of the licensed plasma products are currently nanofiltered. The technology has major advantages as it is flexible and it may combine efficient and largely predictable removal of more than 4 to 6 logs of a wide range of viruses, with an absence of denaturing effect on plasma proteins. Compared with other viral reduction means, nanofiltration may be the only method to date permitting efficient removal of enveloped and non-enveloped viruses under conditions where 90-95% of protein activity is recovered. New data indicate that nanofiltration may also remove prions, opening new perspectives in the development and interest of this technique.

Nanotechnology for point-of-care diagnostics

Point-of-care (POC) or near patient testing means that diagnosis is performed in the doctor's office or at the bed side in case of hospitalized patients or in the field for several other indications including screening of populations for genetic disorders and cancer. POC involves analytical patient testing activities provided within the healthcare system, but performed outside the physical facilities of the clinical laboratories. POC does not require permanent dedicated space but includes kits and instruments, which are either hand carried or transported to the vicinity of the patient for immediate testing at that site. The patients may even conduct the tests. After the laboratory and the emergency room, the most important application of molecular diagnostics is estimated to be at the POC. Nanotechnology would be another means of integrating diagnostics with therapeutics. Nanotechnology-based diagnostics provides the means to monitor drugs administered by nanoparticle carriers.

A number of devices based on nanotechnology are among those with potential applications in POC testing. A method of DNA detection that uses gold nanoparticle probes and microarrays of electrodes has been described (Park et al 2002). It's 10 times more sensitive (causing fewer false negatives) and 100,000 times more selective (causing far fewer false positives) than current methods. The nanoprobes are coated with a synthesized string of nucleotides that complement one end of a target sequence in the sample being analyzed, so they can "grab" it if it's there. Another set of nucleotides, complementing the other end of the target, is attached to a surface between two electrodes. If the target sequence is present in the sample, it attaches to both the nanoprobes and the sequences on the surface between the electrodes, so that the nanoprobes are anchored to the surface like a cluster of little balloons. When they're treated with a silver solution, they create a bridge between the electrodes and produce a charge. The technology could theoretically be used to detect any disease or condition with a unique genomic fingerprint. For example, it could differentiate between various antibiotic-resistant strains of streptococci, or detect cancerous cells, or quickly identify HIV or biological weapons agents like anthrax. A single chip could contain electrode pairs to test for thousands of biological targets at once. And because an electrical charge is either present or absent, there's no ambiguity in the results. Nanosphere Inc's Verigene™ platform will be suitable for development of POC testing.

Detection of infectious agents

The rapid and sensitive detection of pathogenic bacteria is extremely important in medical diagnosis and measures against bioterrorism. Limitations of most of the conventional diagnostic methods are lack ultrasensitivity or delay in getting results. Several nanotechnology based methods have already been described in this chapter including ferrofluid magnetic nanoparticles, ceramic nanospheres and nanowire sensors for viruses. A bioconjugated nanoparticle-based bioassay for in situ pathogen quantification can detect a single bacterium within 20 minutes (Zhao et al 2004). The nanoparticle provides an extremely high fluorescent signal for bioanalysis and can be easily incorporated in a biorecognition molecule such as an antibody. The antibody-conjugated nanoparticles can readily and specifically identify a variety of bacteria such as *Escherichia coli O157:H7* through antibody-antigen interaction and recognition. This method can be applied to multiple bacterial samples with high throughput by using a 384-well microplate format. It has a potential for application in ultrasensitive detection of disease markers and infectious agents.

Detection of bacteria

The technique called SEnsing of Phage-Triggered Ion Cascade (SEPTIC) uses a nanowell device with two antenna-like electrodes to detect the electric-field fluctuations that result when a bacteriophage infects a specific bacterium and then identify the bacterium (Dobozi-King et al 2005). This technology had a 100% success rate in detecting and identifying strains of *E. coli* quickly and accurately. The technique works because only a specific phage can infect a specific bacterium. When a bacteriophage infects a bacterium, the phage injects its DNA into the bacterium and "reprograms" it to produce multiple copies of the phage, called virons. During the infection process, about 100 million ions escape from the host cell. This ion leakage causes fluctuations in the electric field around the bacterium, and the nanowell detects these fluctuations.

Rapid and sensitive identification of bacteria is extremely important in clinical, veterinary and agricultural practice, as well as in applications to microbiological threat detection and reduction. It will also be useful in the current fight against bioterrorism. Eventually, every medic or soldier may be equipped with a cell phone-like, wireless SEPTIC biolab. The researchers' ultimate aim is to have a biochip where hundreds of nanowells and their preamplifiers are integrated. Each nanowell covers a different phage, and if a relevant bacterium is present, the corresponding nanowell will signal and identify the bacterium. This would be a pen-size biolab that would be able to identify hundreds of bacteria in five minutes.

Detection of single virus particles

Microfabrication and application of arrays of silicon cantilever beams as microresonator sensors with nanoscale thickness has been applied to detect the mass of individual virus particles (Gupta et al 2004). The dimensions of the fabricated cantilever beams were in the range of 4–5 μm in length, 1–2 μm in width and 20–30 nm in thickness. The virus particles used in the study were vaccinia virus, which is a member of the Poxviridae family and forms the basis of the smallpox vaccine. The frequency spectra of the cantilever beams, due to thermal and ambient noise, were measured using a laser Doppler vibrometer under ambient conditions. The change in resonant frequency as a function of the virus particle mass binding on the cantilever beam surface forms the basis of the detection scheme. This device can detect a single vaccinia virus particle with an average mass of 9.5 fg. Such devices can be very useful as components of biosensors for the detection of airborne virus particles.

Fluorescent QD probes for detection of respiratory viral infections

Respiratory syncytial virus (RSV) causes about one million deaths annually worldwide. RSV mediates serious lower respiratory tract illness in infants and young children and is a significant pathogen of the elderly and immune compromised. Although it is only life-threatening in one case out of every 100, it infects virtually all children by the time they are five year old. Approximately 120,000 children are hospitalized with RSV in the US each year. Few children in the US die from RSV but it causes 17,000 to 18,000 deaths annually among the elderly.

Rapid and sensitive RSV diagnosis is important for infection control and efforts to develop antiviral drugs. Current RSV detection methods are limited by sensitivity and/or time required for detection, which can take two to six days. This can delay effective treatment. Antibody-conjugated nanoparticles rapidly and sensitively detect RSV and estimate relative levels of surface protein expression (Agrawal et al 2005). A major development is use of dual-color quantum dots (QDs) or fluorescence energy transfer nanobeads that can be simultaneously excited with a single light source.

A QD system can detect the presence of particles of the RSV in a matter of hours. It is also more sensitive, allowing it to detect the virus earlier in the course of an infection (Bentzen et al 2005). When an RSV virus infects lung cells, it leaves part of its coat containing F and G proteins on the cell's surface. QDs have been linked to antibodies keyed to structures unique to RSV's coat. As a result, when QDs come in contact with either viral particles or infected cells they stick to their surface. In addition, co-localization of these viral proteins was shown using confocal microscopy (Figure 7-1).

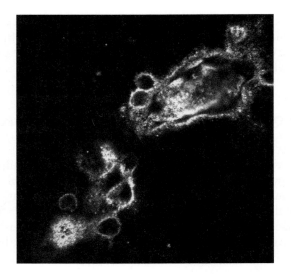

Figure 7-1: Detection of respiratory syncytial virus by quantum dots

A confocal microscope image showing quantum dots that are attached to different antibodies linking two unique structures on the surface of an infected cell.

The potential benefits for such an early detection system for detection of RSV are are that it can:

1. Increase the proper use of antiviral medicines. Although such medicines have been developed for some respiratory viruses, they are not used often as therapy because they are only effective if given early in the course of infection. By the time current tests identify the virus, it is generally too late for them to work.

2. Reduce the inappropriate use of antibiotics. Currently, physicians often prescribe antibiotics for respiratory illnesses. However, antibiotics combat respiratory illness caused by bacteria and are ineffective on viral infections. An early virus detection method would reduce the frequency with which doctors prescribe antibiotics for viral infections inappropriately, thereby reducing unnecessary antibiotic side-effects and cutting down on the development of antibiotic-resistance in bacteria.

3. Allow hospital personnel to isolate RSV patients. RSV is extremely infectious so early detection would allow hospital personnel to keep the RSV patients separate from other patients who are especially susceptible to infection, such as those undergoing bone-marrow transplants.

Currently, there are three diagnostic tests available for identifying respiratory viruses like RSV. The "gold standard" involves incubating an infected sample in a tissue culture for five days and then using a fluorescent dye to test for the presence of the virus. The main problem with this technique is that the virus is multiplying in the patient at the same time as it is growing in the culture. This has caused many hospitals to switch to real time PCR, which is extremely sensitive but still takes 36 to 48 hours because of the need for a technician well trained in molecular biologist to conduct the test in a reference laboratory. The third method, the antigen test, takes only 30 minutes but it is not sensitive enough to detect the presence of the virus at the early stages of an infection. By comparison, the new quantum dot method takes one to two hours and is even more sensitive than real time PCR. It can detect the presence of RSV within an hour after the virus is added to a culture. Another advantage of the QD method over detection systems that rely on fluorescent protein is that the protein "bleaches out" in minutes while QDs maintain their brightness for hours.

It is estimated that it will take only two to three years to develop and validate the QD test. All the components are available off-the-shelf and any one can put together one of these detection system. The system should also be relatively inexpensive. The most costly ingredient is the quantum dots: a small bottle that contains enough of the material for about 200 tests costs $300. As a result, this could be one of the earliest medical applications of nanotechnology. The next step will be to develop a QD cocktail capable of simultaneously detecting the presence of at least five major respiratory viruses: influenza A and B, parainfluenza and metapneumovirus, in addition to RSV. This should be possible because one can use different colors of QDs simultaneously. The colored QDs are attached to different "linker" molecules that bind to different RSV surface structures.QDs are available in a dozen different colors, and antibodies specific to the other four respiratory viruses have been identified and can be used as linker molecules. Such a test would be able to diagnose more than 90% percent of all the cases of viral respiratory infection. The existence of such a test could encourage the development of improved therapies for respiratory viruses. Without a good diagnostic test for a specific viral infection, pharmaceutical companies are not motivated to develop effective treatments because physicians are unlikely to prescribe them very often.

In vivo molecular imaging by use of nanoparticles

There is rapid growth in the use of MRI for molecular and cellular imaging. Much of this work relies on the high relaxivity of nanometer-sized, ultrasmall dextran-coated iron oxide particles. Magnetic nanoparticles, quantum dots and ferrofluids are examples of some of the nanoparticles that have been used along with imaging technologies. Some of the examples are described here.

Superparamagnetic nanoparticles combined with MRI

Highly lymphotropic superparamagnetic nanoparticles measuring 2 to 3 nm on average, which gain access to lymph nodes by means of interstitial-lymphatic fluid transport, have been used in conjunction with high-resolution magnetic resonance imaging (MRI) to reveal small and otherwise undetectable lymph-node metastases (Harisinghani et al 2003). The lymphotropic superparamagnetic nanoparticle used in this study was a monocrystalline iron oxide (Combidex, Advanced Magnetics). In patients with prostate cancer who underwent surgical lymph-node resection or biopsy, MRI with lymphotropic superparamagnetic nanoparticles correctly identified all patients with nodal metastases. This diagnosis was not possible with conventional MRI alone and has implications for the management. In men with metastatic prostate cancer, adjuvant androgen-deprivation therapy with radiation is the mainstay of management.

The presence of lymph node metastases is an important factor in breast cancer patient prognosis. Therefore, the precise identification of sentinel lymph nodes in these patients is critical. Draining lymphatic ducts and lymph nodes were clearly visualized in the mammary tissue of normal mice and in spontaneous and xenografted breast tumor models after a direct mammary gland or peritumoral injection of nano-size paramagnetic molecule, G6. Micro-magnetic resorance lymphangiography using the G6 contrast agent revealed the absence of filling in the metastatic foci of affected lymph nodes (Kobayashi et al 2004). Gd-DTPA-dime-glumine, by contrast, failed to depict lymphatic flow from the mammary tissue in normal mice using the same method. The superior temporal and spatial resolution of micro-MR lymphangiography using the contrast agent G6 may facilitate the study of tumor lymphatic drainage and lymphatic metastasis in both experimental animals and clinical medicine. In addition, this may be a powerful new method for sentinel lymph node localization in human breast cancer.

Ultrasmall superparamagnetic iron oxide (USPIO) as a cell-specific contrast agent for MRI An open-label phase II study has tested the potential of USPIO-enhanced MRI for macrophage imaging in human ischemic lesions (Saleh et al 2004). USPIO-induced signal alterations throughout differed from signatures of conventional gadolinium-enhanced MRI, thus being independent from breakdown of the blood-brain barrier. Macrophages, as the prevailing inflammatory cell population in stroke, contribute to brain damage. USPIO-enhanced MRI may provide an in vivo surrogate marker of cellular inflammation in stroke and other CNS pathologies. USPIO has favorable properties that result from its intravascular retention and lack of extravasation, allowing optimal contrast between the vessel and the adjacent tissue for several minutes postinjection (Corot et al 2003). SH U 555 C (Schering AG) is an optimized formulation of carboxydextran-coated ferucarbotran (Schering's Resovist) is another USPIO. When injected as a bolus at highest dose of 40 micromol Fe/kg, it has capability for depiction at first-pass magnetic resonance angiography and for cardiac perfusion (Reimer et al 2004).

Nanoparticles as contrast agent for MRI

The determination of brain tumor margins both during the presurgical planning phase and during surgical resection has long been a challenging task in the therapy of brain tumor patients. Multimodal (near-infrared fluorescent and magnetic) nanoparticles were used as a preoperative magnetic resonance imaging contrast agent and intraoperative optical probe in a model of gliosarcoma with stably green fluorescence protein-expressing 9L glioma cells (Kircher et al 2003). Key features of nanoparticle metabolism, namely intracellular sequestration by microglia and the combined optical and magnetic properties of the probe, allowed delineation of brain tumors both by preoperative MRI and by intraoperative optical imaging. This prototypical multimodal nanoparticle has unique properties that may allow radiologists and neurosurgeons to see the same probe in the same cells and may offer a new approach for obtaining tumor margins.

An iron oxide nanoparticle can outline not only brain tumors under MRI but also other lesions in the brain that may otherwise have gone unnoticed (Neuwelt et al 2004). Ferumoxtran-10 (Combidex®, Advanced Magnetics Inc), a dextran-coated iron oxide nanoparticle, provides enhancement of intracranial tumors by MRI for more than 24 h and can be imaged histologically by iron staining. Each iron oxide nanoparticle is the size of a small virus and is much smaller than a bacterium but much larger than an atom or standard gadolinium contrast molecule. It's an iron oxide crystal surrounded with a carbohydrate or 'sugar' coating called dextran, which gives the particle a longer plasma half-life, allowing it to slowly slip through the blood-brain barrier – a natural defense system that blocks the entry of foreign substances, including therapeutic agents.

Quantum dots for biological imaging

Accurate imaging of diseased cells (e.g., primary and metastatic tumors) is of primary importance in disease management. The National Institutes of Health (NIH) has developed carbohydrate-encapsulated quantum dots (QDs) with detectable luminescent properties useful for imaging of cancer or other disease tissues. Certain carbohydrates, especially those included on tumor glycoproteins are known to have affinity for certain cell types. One notable glycan used in this technology is the Thomsen-Freidenreich disaccharide (Galbeta1-3GalNAc) that is readily detectable in 90% of all primary human carcinomas and their metastases. These glycans can be exploited for medical imaging. Encapsulating luminescent QDs with target- specific glycans permits efficient imaging of the tissue to which the glycans bind with high affinity.

Multifunctional nanoparticle probes based on semiconductor QDs have been used for cancer targeting and imaging in living animals. The structural design involves encapsulating luminescent QDs with an ABC triblock copolymer and linking this amphiphilic polymer to tumor-targeting ligands and drug-delivery functionalities. In vivo targeting studies of human prostate cancer growing in nude mice indicate that the QD probes accumulate at tumors both by the enhanced permeability and retention of tumor sites and by antibody binding to cancer-specific cell surface biomarkers (Gao et al 2004). Using both subcutaneous injection of QD-tagged cancer cells and systemic injection of multifunctional QD, sensitive and multicolor fluorescence imaging of cancer cells have been achieved under in vivo conditions. These results raise new possibilities for ultrasensitive and multiplexed imaging of molecular targets in vivo.

Nanoparticles vs microparticles for cellular imaging

Typically, millions of dextran-coated ultrasmall iron oxide particles (USIOPs) must be loaded into cells for efficient detection. A recent study shows that single, micrometer-sized iron oxide particles (MPIOPs) can be detected by MRI in vitro in agarose samples, in cultured cells, and in mouse embryos (Shapiro et al 2004). Experiments studying effects of MRI resolution and particle size from indicated that significant signal effects could be detected at resolutions as low as 200 μm. Cultured cells were labeled with fluorescent MPIOPs such that single particles were present in individual cells. These single particles in single cells could be detected both by MRI and fluorescence microscopy. Finally, single particles injected into single-cell-stage mouse embryos could be detected at later embryonic stages, demonstrating that even after many cell divisions, daughter cells still carry individual particles. These results demonstrate that MRI can detect single particles and indicate that single-particle detection will be useful for cellular imaging for certain purposes and may be preferable to nanoparticles. MPIOPs will useful in following the division of stem cells and in vivo labeling of cells.

Nano-endoscopy

NanoRobotics Laboratory at the Carnegie-Mellon University (CMU, Pittsburgh, PA) is developing endoscopic microcapsules that can be ingested and precisely positioned. A control system will allow the capsule to attach to the digestive tract and move within the digestive. Several different methods are being researched for the attachment of microcapsules including both dry and wet adhesion as well as mechanical methods such as a set of tripod legs with adhesive on feet. A simple model with surface characteristics similar to that of the digestive tract will be constructed to test these methods.

Precisely positioned microcapsules would allow doctors to view any part of the inside lining of the digestive tract in detail resulting in more efficient, accurate, and less invasive diagnoses. In addition, these capsules could be modified to include treatment mechanisms as well, such as the release of a drug or chemical near an abnormal area.

Given Imaging Ltd (Yoqneam, Israel) pioneered imaging capsules. Its PillCam™ capsule endoscope, a tool to visualize small intestine abnormalities, was approved in 2001. Other companies are now producing ingestible capsules for this purpose. The patient ingests the capsule, which contains a tiny camera and intestinal peristalsis propels the capsule for approximately eight hours. During this time, the camera snaps the pictures and images that are transmitted to a data recorder worn by the patient. The physicians can review the images later on to make the diagnosis but some abnormalities may be missed as this method has only a 50% success rate in detection of diseases. Controlling the positioning and movement on a nanoscale will greatly improve the accuracy of this method.

The so called "gutbot" in development at CMU is based on nanotechnology including nanosensors and sticking devices. If this device is successful, its use may be extended to the large intestine.

Although colon is currently examined by colonoscopy, physicians might be interested in introducing a pill-sized camera through the anus to visualize the suspicious area.Similar nanorobots are under development for other parts of the body.

Nanodiagnostics for the development of personalized medicine

Molecular diagnostics is an important component of personalized medicine. Improvement of diagnostics by nanotechnology has a positive impact on personalized medicine. Nanotechnology has potential advantages in applications in point-of-care (POC) diagnosis: on patient's bedside, self-diagnostics for use in the home and integration of diagnostics with therapeutics. All of these will facilitate the development of personalized medicines.

8. COMMERCIAL ASPECTS OF NANOMOLECULAR DIAGNOSTICS

Abstract

Markets for in vitro diagnostic applications of nanobiotechnology are estimated to reach a value of $1billion in 2005, $2.5 billion in 2010 and $9.5 billion in 2015. The related market of imaging applications of nanotechnology is estimated at $0.5 billion for 2005, $1.25 billion for 2010 and $5 billion for 2015. These figures include developments in both the academic and commercial sectors.

Introduction

Markets for nanomolecular diagnostics are difficult to estimate because they overlap with markets for molecular diagnostic technologies and nanobiotechnology. In the year 2005, the global market for molecular diagnostics will be worth $6.5 billion, representing approximately 3.3% of the total diagnostics market and approximately 14% of the in vitro diagnostic market. The molecular diagnostics market will expand to $12 billion by 2010 and $35 billion by 2015. A major portion of expansion in molecular diagnostics can be attributed to advances in genomics and proteomics. Biochip and nanobiotechnology are expected to make a significant contribution to the growth of molecular diagnostics. The shift from clinical to molecular diagnostics, emphasis on preventive medicine, integration of diagnostics with therapeutics and development of personalized medicine will drive the growth of molecular diagnostics.

Markets for nanomolecular diagnostics

It is more difficult to calculate market potential of nanobiotechnology than that of molecular diagnostics. Based on a review of the current status and future potential, nanobiotechnologies can be expected to grow to $8 billion in 2005, $20 billion in 2010 and $70 billion in 2015. This tremendous jump from 2010-2015 is due to the development of nanobiotechnologies that will replace many of the current technologies. This is not calculated on any percentage growth but based on the anticipated state of development of nanobiotechnology by the year 2015.

Markets for in vitro diagnostic applications of nanobiotechnology are estimated to reach a value of $1.00 billion in 2005, $2.50 billion in 2010 and $09.50 billion in 2015. The related market of imaging applications of nanotechnology is estimated at $0.50 billion for 2005, $1.25 billion for 20110 and $05.00 billion for 2015. These figures include developments in both the academic and commercial sectors. An idea of the commercial sector can be obtained by the companies involved in nanomolecular diagnostics and their products.

Companies involved in nanomolecular diagnostics

Selected companies/laboratories involved in nanomolecular diagnostics are shown in Table 8-1.

Table 8-1: Companies developing nanomolecular diagnostics

Company/Laboratory	Technology	Applications
Acrongenomics Inc (Calgary, Canada)	Neo-EpCAM™ Detection Kit based on Nano-JETA™ Real Time PCR	Early diagnosis of epithelial cancers e.g., involving the gastrointestinal tract
Advance Nanotech Inc (New York, NY)	Bionanosensors that can be implanted within the body	To diagnose and treat a wide variety of medical conditions
Advanced Magnetics Inc (Cambridge, MA)	Combidex®, an investigational iron oxide nanoparticle combined with MRI	Non-invasive evaluation of lymph nodes in patients with prostate cancer
Agilent Laboratories (Palo Alto, CA)	Nanopore technology that converts strings of nucleotides directly into electronic signatures.	Cost-effective and quick sequencing of individual, chromosome-length molecules of DNA
Agilent Technologies /Caliper (Palo Alto, CA)	RNA 6000 Nano LabChip kit	For the automated quality control of total and messenger RNA
AION Diagnostics (Perth, Australia)	Diagnostic and sensor applications of the BioSilicon™ platform technology	To provide real time continuous measurement of diagnostic markers
Ambri Ltd (Chatswood, Australia)	Ion Channel Switch (ICS™)-based integrates biotechnology, nanotechnology and electronics	The product – SensiDx™ System – has been designed for POC testing in critical care environments in hospitals
Arryx Inc (Chicago, IL)	BioRyx® 200 system: laser tweezers to manipulate nanoscopic objects	Nanosensor as a diagnostics tool to spot chemicals and biological agents

Ayanda Biosystems (Lausanne, Switzerland)	Synthetic ligand-gated ion channel biosensor that can detect biomolecules	Diagnosis of infectious diseases
BioForce Nanosciences (Ames, IA)	Ultra-miniaturized nanoarray technologies for biomolecular analysis	Disease diagnosis and biowarfare agent detection system
BioNanomatrix (Princeton, NJ)	NanoImprinting Lithography used to fabricated millions of nanofluidic structures with very small dimensions	For analysis of long genomic DNA and scan for the medically relevant bound genetical markers
Biophan Technologies (West Henrietta, NY)	Contrast agent with nanomagnetic particles (NanoView) that would be swallowed or injected	For improved MRI testing and safe use in those with implanted metal devices
BioPixels (Westerville, OH)	BioPixels™ are semiconductor-based, fluorescent nanocrystalline particles	Fluorescence-based detection assays: immunofluorescence, Western blot, etc
Cantion A/S (Lyngby, Copenhagen)	Cantilever technology	Detection of microorganisms and biowarfare agents
Chemicon International Inc (Temecula, CA)	Quantum dot-containing products	Detection of antibody-antigen interactions
Concentris GmbH (Basel, Switzerland)	Cantilever technology	Detection of DNA, proteins and microorganisms
Crystalplex Corporation (Pittsburgh, PA)	CrystalBeads (quantum dot microbeads) assays for biomolecules	SNP profiling, protein interaction studies, and clinical diagnostics
EngeneOS Inc (Waltham, MA)	DNA nanomachines	Biomolecular detectors for homogeneous assays
Evident Technologies (Troy, NY)	EviArrays biochips based on nanocystal technology	To detect microorganisms such as anthrax and smallpox
Hitachi Co Ltd (Tokyo, Japan)	A silicon "stamp" that presses onto a polystyrene-based polymer film, producing nanopillars on a chip	Ultrasensitive detectors Drug discovery
IBM (Zurich, Switzerland)	Microcantilever technology	Can detect single base pair changes in DNA
Integrated Nanosystems Inc (Los Gatos, CA)	NESA™ (Nano Electrode Sensor Array) chip	Biosensor for detection of DNA and microorganisms
Integrated Nano-Technologies (Henrietta, NY)	BioDetect™ is a detection device based on integration of DNA and electronics	A portable biological agent detector
Immunicon Corporation (Huntingdon Valley, PA)	CellTracks™ based on Ferrofluids – magnetic nanoparticles for isolating cells from complex biological mixtures	Diagnosis of circulating cells in cancer
Invitrogen (San Diego, CA)	Genicon's Resonance Light Scattering technology relies on nanoparticles	SNP analysis, DNA/RNA probes Antigen/antibody assays
Lawrence Berkeley National Laboratory (Berkeley, CA)	The smallest laser—a nanowire nanolaser	Chemical analysis on microchips

Luna Innovations (Blacksburg, VA)	Trimetaspheres: soccer-ball shaped nanomolecules made of pure carbon	Increase the sensitivity of MRI scans Identify and attack cancer cells
Maxwell Sensors Inc (Santa Fe Springs, CA)	A wavelength coded quantum bead technology for multiple analyte assays	All-in-one disease diagnostics Cell analysis
Molecular Nanosystems (Palo Alto, CA)	Miniature chemical and biological sensors based on carbon nanotubes	Environmental monitoring, military, medical and biotechnology applications
NanoBiomics Inc/ Molecular Profiling Institute (Phoenix, AZ)	Genomics-based diagnostics using nanoscale processing technologies	Molecular diagnostics Personalized medicine
NanoCarrier Co Ltd (Chiba, Japan)	NanoCoat technology is used in a new ELISA system	Immunodiagnostics
NanoWave Inc (Lynn, MA)	NanoWave Scanning Probe Position Encoder	Medical diagnostics
NanoInk (Chicago, IL)	Dip Pen Nanolithography™ technology for ultra-miniaturization of DNA arrays	Point-of-care diagnostics and biodefense
Nanogen Inc (San Diego, CA)	NanoChip Molecular Biology Workstation to bridge research and clinical diagnostics	To provide quick and accurate analysis of DNA, RNA and proteins
Nanomagnetics (Bristol, UK)	Magnetoferritin: magnetic particles in protein spheres – 12 nm in diameter	MRI contrast enhancement agent
Nanomix Inc (Emeryville, CA)	Single-walled carbon nanotubes in nanosensors are only one molecular layer thick and extremely sensitive	Biological detection, including blood gas monitoring, protein assays, and pathogen detection
Nanoparticles Co Ltd (Chiba, Japan)	Micellar nanoparticles bound with antibodies	Immunodiagnostic reagents
Nanoplex Technologies (Menlo Park, CA)	Nanobarcodes are cylindrical metal nanoparticles that vary the composition along the particle length	Enables multiplexed bioanalytical measurements in microvolume samples. Used as identification tags.
Nanoprobes Inc (Yaphank, NY)	Nanogold®: gold labels are uncharged molecules which are cross-linked to specific sites on biomolecules	These labels can be attached to any molecule with a reactive group - proteins, peptides, oligonucleotides, small molecules and lipids - for detection and localization
NanoSight Ltd (Salisbury, UK)	Halo™LM10: attachment to an existing optical microscope can be used to visualize nanoscale particles	Detection of viruses and DNA
Nanospectra Biosciences (Houston, Texas)	Nanoshells may be used in immunoassays	Rapid, quantitative results in a fraction of the time required by current ELISA
Nanosphere Inc (Northbrook, IL)	Nanoparticle probes based on gold nanoparticles	SNP genotyping and genomic DNA detection

NanoString Technologies (Seattle, WA)	Nanotechnology-based platform for automated high speed, single molecule identification and digital quantification	Gene expression analysis Molecular diagnostics/ genotyping Proteomics
Nanosys Inc (Palo Alto, CA)	An exquisitely sensitive and flexible molecular sensing system that utilizes a tiny nanowire, decorated with specific capture molecules	Detects the presence of minute quantities of analytes such as ions, nucleic acids and proteins
Nanotype (Munich, Germany)	Nanoscale balance to measure unbinding forces between single biomolecules	Molecular diagnostics
Nomadics Inc (Stillwater, OK, USA)	Photostimulated luminescence in nanoparticles, which emit light in on exposure to various types of energy	In vivo imaging probes
NVE Corporation (Eden Prairie, MN)	BioMagnetIC ultra-miniature biosensors	Biological warfare agent detectors Laboratory-on-a-chip diagnostics
OraSure Technologies (Bethlehem, PA)	Up-Converting Phosphor Technology: ceramic nanospheres composed of rare earth metals are 1000 times more sensitive than fluorescent technologies	Drug discovery, SNP analysis, and infectious disease testing
Oxonica (Oxfordshire, UK)	Surface-Enhanced Resonant Raman Spectroscopy and Nanocrystals	Ultrasensitive, high throughput diagnostics
PharmaSeq Inc (Monmouth Junction,NJ)	Light-powered microtransponders and nanotransponders	DNA probe diagnostics, SNP detection, and proteomics
Protiveris Inc (Rockville, MD)	Technology based on chemo-mechanical actuation of specially designed silicon microcantilevers and subsequent optical detection of deflections	Microcantilever arrays provide the potential to make this technique superior to existing biosensor technologies for diagnostics.
Quantum Dot Corporation (Hayward, CA)	Qdot nanocrystals are photostable and water-soluble. They light up in selected colors when exposed to ultraviolet light	Qdot assays can be used for immunocytochemistry, Western/dot blotting, microarrays and FISH
Quantum Magnetics Inc (San Diego, CA)	Quadrupole resonance, magnetic resonance and electromagnetic sensing	Magnetic sensor to detect excessive amount of iron in liver
Solex (Little Chesterford, UK)	Single Molecule Array nanotechnology for the independent analysis of a billion individual DNA molecules in parallel	Study of genetic variation and development of personalized medicine
Spinelix (Saint Beauzire, France)	Biological analysis, protein and DNA microarrays, capillary electrophoresis	Sequencing and tagged/ untagged molecule detection
Xeptagen (Marghera, Italy)	Cancer polymarker biochip: nanosized opto-electronic sensing device	Detection of biomarkers for early detection of cancer

9. CONCLUDING REMARKS & FUTURE PROSPECTS OF NANODIAGNOSTICS

Abstract

It is concluded that direct analysis of DNA and protein could dramatically improve speed, accuracy, and sensitivity over conventional molecular diagnostic methods. The potential of single molecule analysis approach would not be fully realized without the help of nanobiotechnology. Nanodiangostics would provide a completely detailed "snapshot" of cellular, subcellular and molecular activities. Such a detailed diagnosis would guide the appropriate treatment.

Concluding remarks

It is now obvious that direct analysis of DNA and protein could dramatically improve speed, accuracy, and sensitivity over conventional molecular diagnostic methods. Since DNA, RNA, protein and their functional subcellular scaffolds and compartments, are in the nanometer scale, the potential of single molecule analysis approach would not be fully realized without the help of nanobiotechnology. Advances in nanotechnology are providing nanofabricated devices that are small, sensitive and inexpensive enough to facilitate direct observation, manipulation and analysis of single biological molecule from single cell. This opens new opportunities and provides powerful tools in the fields such as genomics, proteomics, molecular diagnostics and high throughput screening.

Within the next decade, measurement devices based on nanotechnology, which can make thousands of measurements very rapidly and very inexpensively, will become available. The most common clinical diagnostic application will be blood protein analysis. Blood in systemic circulation reflects the state of health or disease of most organs. Therefore, detection of blood molecular fingerprints will provide a sensitive assessment of health and disease.

Various nanodiagnostics that have been reviewed will improve the sensitivity and extend the present limits of molecular diagnostics. Numerous nanodevices and nanosystems for sequencing single molecules of DNA are feasible. It seems quite likely that there will be numerous applications of inorganic nanostructures in biology and medicine as markers. Given the inherent nanoscale of receptors, pores, and other functional components of living cells, the detailed monitoring and analysis of these components will be made possible by the development of a new class of nanoscale probes. Biological tests measuring the presence or activity of selected substances become quicker, more sensitive and more flexible when certain nanoscale particles are put to work as tags or labels. Nanoparticles are the most versatile material for developing diagnostics.

Nanomaterials can be assembled into massively parallel arrays at much higher densities than is achievable with current sensor array platforms and in a format compatible with current microfluidic systems. Currently, quantum dot technology is the most widely employed nanotechnology for diagnostic developments. Among the recently emerging technologies, cantilevers are the most promising. This technology complements and extends current DNA and protein microarray methods, because nanomechanical detection requires no labels, optical excitation, or external probes and is rapid, highly specific, sensitive, and portable. This will have applications in genomic analysis, proteomics and molecular diagnostics. Nanosensors are promising for detection of bioterrorism agents that are not detectable with current molecular diagnostic technologies and some have already been developed.

Future prospects of nanodiagnostics

In the near future, nanodiagnostics would reduce the waiting time for the test results. For example, the patients with sexually transmitted diseases could give the urine sample when they first arrive at the outpatient clinic or physician's practice; the results could then be ready by the time they go in to see the doctor. They could then be given the prescription immediately, reducing the length of time worrying for the patient and making the whole process cheaper.

Future trends in diagnostics will continue in miniaturization of biochip technology to nano range. There is also a trend to build the diagnostic devices from bottom up starting with the smallest building blocks. Whether interest and application of nanomechanical detection will hold in the long range remains to be seen. Another trend is to move away from fluorescent labeling as miniaturization reduces the signal intensity but there have been some improvements making fluorescent viable with nanoparticles. Current research projects at academic centers that are relevant to nanodiagnostics are listed in Table 9-1.

Table 9-1: Academic institutes/laboratories involved in nanomolecular diagnostics

Center/program	Parent Institutes	Areas of interest
Applied NanoBioscience	The Biodesign Institute, State University of Arizona (Tempe, AZ)	To develop biological tools based on nanoscale technologies to understand disease at the molecular level
Biomedical Engineering Center	Industrial Technology Research Institute (Taiwan)	In vivo nanodevices, biomimetic sensing, nanobiolabeling/diagnosis
Bio-molecular Engineering Group	University of Missouri (Columbia, MO)	Engineered membrane protein channels used to make single molecule biosensors
BioSecurity and NanoSciences Laboratory	Lawrence Livermore National Laboratory (Livermore, CA)	Nanoscience to detect even the single smallest molecule of harmful substances
California Nanosystems Institute	UCLA, Univ of California (Santa Barbara), industry and the state of California	Molecular-level diagnosis and treatment of disease
Center for Biologic Nanotechnology	University of Michigan (Ann Arbor, MI)	Dendrimers Nanoemulsions
Center for Molecular Imaging Research	Massachusetts General Hospital (Boston, MA)	Nanoparticles for in vivo sensing and imaging of molecular events
Center for Nanotechnology	University of Washington (Seattle, WA)	Bionanotechnology for cancer diagnostics and therapeutics
Center for Nanotechnology	NASA Ames Research Center (Moffett Field, CA)	Carbon nanotubes and nanowires for biological sensing
Cornell NanoScale Science & Technology Facility	Cornell University (Ithaca, NY)	Biosensors and microarrays
Center for Nanoscience & Nanotechnology	Georgia Institute of Technology (Atlanta, GA)	Nanodevicies and nanosensors for biotechnology
FIRST (Frontiers in Research, Space and Time)	Swiss Federal Inst of Technol (Zurich, Switzerland)	AFM as a nanolithography tool
Heath Group	California Institute of Technology (Pasadena, CA)	Nanobiology: Nanolab combines several assays on a cm² silicon chip resembling a miniature cell farm with rows of cells
IMTEK - Institute of Microsystem Technology	University of Freiburg, (Freiburg, Germany)	Nanoparticles for biosensors
Institute of NanoScience and Engineering	University of Pittsburgh (Pittsburgh, PA)	Use of nanotubes to create a "nanocarpet" to detect and destroy bacteria

Institute for Nanotechnology	Northwestern University (Evanston, IL)	Nanoparticles and biosensors; nano-bar-code for detection of proteins; nanofibers for neuroregeneration
Institute of Micro- and Nanotechnology	Technical University of Denmark, Denmark	Study of nanoscale structures with in situ scanning tunneling microscopy
Laboratory for Micro- and Nanotechnology	Paul Scherrer Institute (Villigen, Switzerland)	Nanopore membranes, biosensors and artificial noses
Laboratory for Photonics and Nanostructures	CNRS (Marcoussis, France)	Separation methods for DNA sequencing Protein analysis and on-chip detection Microfluidic systems for cell sorting.
Lerner Research Institute	The Cleveland Clinic (Cleveland, OH)	Nanometer-scale tissue engineering, diagnostics, nanosensors for surgery
London Center for Nanotechnology	University College (London, UK)	Use of nanotechnology to develop low cost diagnostics and personalized medicine
National Center for Competence in Research Nanoscale Science	Biozentrum, University of Basel (Basel, Switzerland)	To bring nanotechnology from the bench to the patient by developing new tools
Nano-Biomolecular Engineering Group	University of California (Berkeley, CA)	BioCOM cantilever chip for cancer diagnosis, DNA-based self-assembly/ replication of inorganic nanostructures, and electrophoretic separation microchip
NanoBioTechnology Initiative	Ohio University (Athens, OH)	Diagnosis/treatment: cancer and diabetes
Nanoscale Science and Engineering program	Rice University (Houston, Texas)	Nanobiotechnology: nanoscale sensory systems, biochips.
Roukes Group	California Institute of Technology (Pasadena, CA)	Nanotechnology for neurophysiology Nanodevices for molecular biosensing
Sandia National Laboratories (Albuquerque, NM)	Dept of Energy, US Government	Nanodevices: biosensors to detect biological agents
Winship Cancer Institute	Emory University (Atlanta, GA)	Cancer nanotechnology: nanoparticles for molecular and cellular imaging.

Impact of nanodiagnostics on future of nanomedicine

Nanotechnology will also provide devices to examine tissue in minute detail. Biosensors that are smaller than a cell would give us an inside look at cellular function. Tissues could be analyzed down to the molecular level, giving a completely detailed "snapshot" of cellular, subcellular and molecular activities. Such a detailed diagnosis would guide the appropriate treatment.

It is expected that within the next few years, we will have a better understanding of how to coat or chemically alter nanoparticles to reduce their toxicity to the body, which will allow us to broaden their use for disease diagnosis and for drug delivery. Biomedical applications are likely to be some of the earliest. The first clinical trials are anticipated cancer therapy.

Nanodiagnostics and oncology

Most of the advances in nanodiagnostics are anticipated in oncology. Another important area of application will be cancer diagnostics. Molecular diagnosis of cancer including genetic profiling would be widely used by the year 2015. The use of nanotechnology enables researchers to combine traditional pathology and cancer biology with highly sensitive molecular analysis. Collaborative research is expected to produce a database linking molecular signatures with clinical outcome; a new class of nanoparticles for molecular profiling of cancer; and imaging microscopes and software that are integrated with the new discoveries in nanotechnology. Advanced nanoparticle quantum dot probes will be developed for molecular and cellular imaging. Bioconjugated quantum dots will be chemically linked to molecules such as antibodies, peptides, proteins or DNA and engineered to detect other molecules, such as those present on the surface of cancer cells. A variety of molecules involved in the development and progression of cancer will be studied, including those involved in programmed cell death; genes such as the p53 gene, which is implicated in many kinds of cancer; and microtubules and molecular motors, which are involved in transporting the proteins in cells that regulate cell growth. Nanobiotechnology would play an important part, not only in cancer diagnosis but also in linking diagnosis with treatment.

REFERENCES

Agrawal A, Tripp RA, Anderson LJ, Nie S. Real-time detection of virus particles and viral protein expression with two-color nanoparticle probes. J Virol 2005 Jul;79:8625-8.

Avery OT, McLeod CM, McCarty M. Studies on the chemical nature of the substance inducing transformation of pneumococcal types. Journal of Experimental Medicine 1944;79:137-158.

Bao YP, Huber M, Wei TF, et al. SNP identification in unamplified human genomic DNA with gold nanoparticle probes. Nucleic Acids Res 2005;33:e15.

Barlaan EA, Sugimori M, Furukawa S, Takeuchi K. Electronic microarray analysis of 16S rDNA amplicons for bacterial detection. J Biotechnol 2005;115:11-21.

Barone PW, Baik S, Heller DA, Strano MS. Near-infrared optical sensors based on single-walled carbon nanotubes. Nature Materials 2005;4:86–92.

Batten TF, Hopkins CR. Use of protein A-coated colloidal gold particles for immunoelectronmicroscopic localization of ACTH on ultrathin sections. Histochemistry 1979;60:317-20.

Bayley H, Jayasinghe L. Functional engineered channels and pores. Mol Membrane Biol 2004;21:209-20.

Benenson Y, Gil B, Ben-Dor U, Adar R, Shapiro E. An autonomous molecular computer for logical control of gene expression. Nature 2004;429:423-9.

Bentzen EL, House F, Utley TJ, et al. Progression of respiratory syncytial virus infection monitored by fluorescent quantum dot probes. Nano Lett 2005;5:591-5.

Bietsch A, Zhang J, Hegner M, et al. Rapid functionalization of cantilever array sensors by inkjet printing. Nanotechnology 2004;15:873-880.

Bock LC, Griffin LC, Latham JA, et al. Selection of single-stranded DNA molecules that bind and inhibit human thrombin. Nature 1992;355:564-6.

Borsting C, Sanchez JJ, Morling N. SNP typing on the NanoChip electronic microarray. Methods Mol Biol 2005;297:155-68.

Braydich-Stolle L, Hussain S, Schlager J, Hofmann MC. In vitro cytotoxicity of nanoparticles in mammalian germ-line stem cells. Toxicol Sci 2005 Jul 13; [Epub ahead of print].

Bruchez M Jr, Moronne M, Gin P, Weiss S, Alivisatos AP. Semiconductor nanocrystals as fluorescent biological labels. Science 1998;281:2013-6.

Bruemmel Y, Chan CP, Renneberg R, et al. On the influence of different surfaces in nano- and submicrometer particle based fluorescence immunoassays. Langmuir 2004;20:9371-9.

Bulte JW, Arbab AS, Douglas T, et al. Preparation of magnetically labeled cells for cell tracking by magnetic resonance imaging. Methods Enzymol 2004;386:275-99.

Cai H, Xu Y, Zhu N, He P, Fang Y. An electrochemical DNA hybridization detection assay based on a silver nanoparticle label. Analyst 2002;127:803-8.

Cao H, Tegenfeldt JO, Austin RH, Chou SY. Gradient nanostructures for interfacing microfluidics and nanofluidics Applied Physics Letters 2002a;81:3058–3060.

Cao H, Yu Z, Wang J, et al. Fabrication of 10 nm enclosed nanofluidic channels. Applied Physics Letters 2002;81:174–176.

Cao Y, Lee Koo YE, Kopelman R. Poly(decyl methacrylate)-based fluorescent PEBBLE swarm nanosensors for measuring dissolved oxygen in biosamples. Analyst 2004;129:745-50.

Chang E, Miller JS, Sun J, et al. Protease-activated quantum dot probes. Biochem Biophys Res Commun 2005;334:1317-21.

Chemla YR, Grossman HL, Poon Y, et al. Ultrasensitive magnetic biosensor for homogeneous immunoassay. PNAS 2000;97:14268-72.

Chen RJ, Bangsaruntip S, Drouvalakis KA, et al. Noncovalent functionalization of carbon nanotubes for highly specific electronic biosensors. PNAS 2003;100:4984–4989.

Cherukuri P, Bachilo SM, Litovsky SH, Weisman RB. Near-Infrared Fluorescence Microscopy of Single-Walled Carbon Nanotubes in Phagocytic Cells. J Am Chem Soc 2004;126:15638-15639.

Cornell BA. Optical Biosensors: Present and Future. In, Lighler F, Taitt CR (eds) Membrane based Biosensors. Elsevier, Amsterdam, 2002;Chapter 12: p 457.

Corot C, Violas X, Robert P, Gagneur G, Port M. Comparison of different types of blood pool agents (P792, MS325, USPIO) in a rabbit MR angiography-like protocol. Invest Radiol 2003;38:311-9.

Crut A, Geron-Landre B, Bonnet I, et al. Detection of single DNA molecules by multicolor quantum-dot end-labeling. Nucleic Acids Research 2005;33:e98.

Curl RF, Kroto H, Smalley RE. Nobel lectures in chemistry. Reviews of Modern Physics 1997;69:691-730.

Cutillas PR. Principles of Nanoflow Liquid Chromatography and Applications to Proteomics. Current Nanoscience 2005;1:65-71.

Dahan M, Levi S, Luccardini C, et al. Diffusion dynamics of glycine receptors revealed by single-quantum dot tracking. Science 2003;302:442-5.

Delfino I, Bizzarri AR, Cannistraro S. Single-molecule detection of yeast cytochrome c by Surface-Enhanced Raman Spectroscopy. Biophys Chem 2005;113:41-51.

Denk W, Horstmann H. Serial block-face scanning electron microscopy to reconstruct three-dimensional tissue nanostructure. PLoS Biol 2004;2:e329.

Derfus AM, Chan CW, Bhatia SN, et al. Probing the Cytotoxicity of Semiconductor Quantum Dots Nano Letters 2004;4:11 - 18.

Di Giusto DA, Wlassoff WA, Gooding JJ, et al. Proximity extension of circular DNA aptamers with real-time protein detection. Nucleic Acids Res 2005;33:e64.

Dobozi-King M, Seo S, Kim JU, Young R, Cheng M, Kish L. Rapid Detection and Identification of Bacteria: SEnsing of Phage-Triggered Ion Cascade (SEPTIC). Journal of Biological Physics and Chemistry 2005;5:3-7.

Douglas SJ, Davis SS, Illum L. Nanoparticles in drug delivery. Crit Rev Ther Drug Carrier Syst. 1987;3:233-61.

Downs ME, Warner PJ, Turner AP, Fothergill JC. Optical and electrochemical detection of DNA. Biomaterials 1988;9:66-70.

Drexler KE. Engines of creation, the coming era of nanotechnology. Anchor, New York, 1987.

Ebner A, Kienberger F, Kada G, et al. Localization of single avidin-biotin interactions using simultaneous topography and molecular recognition imaging. Chemphyschem 2005;6:897-900.

Eigler DM, Schweizer EK. Positioning single atoms with a scanning tunneling nicroscope. Nature 1990;344:524-6.

El-Sayed IH, Huang X, El-Sayed MA. Surface Plasmon Resonance Scattering and Absorption of anti-EGFR Antibody Conjugated Gold Nanoparticles in Cancer Diagnostics: Applications in Oral Cancer. Nano Lett 2005;5:829-834.

Englebienne P, Van Hoonacker A, Verhas M, Khlebtsov NG. Advances in high-throughput screening: biomolecular interaction monitoring in real-time with colloidal metal nanoparticles. Comb Chem High Throughput Screen. 2003;6:777-87.

Fang N, Lee H, Sun C, Zhang X. Sub–Diffraction-Limited Optical Imaging with a Silver Superlens. Science 2005;308: 534-537.

Farrer RA, Butterfield FL, Chen VW, Fourkas JT. Highly Efficient Multiphoton-Absorption-Induced Luminescence from Gold Nanoparticles. Nano Lett 2005: 1139-42.

Feynman R. There's plenty of room at the bottom: an invitation to enter a new filed of physics. Reprinted in: Crandall BC, Lewis J (eds) Nanotechnology: research and perspectives. The MIT Press, Cambridge, MA, 1992:347-363.

Fodor SP, Read JL, Pirrung MC, et al. Light-directed, spatially addressable parallel chemical synthesis. Science 1991;251:763-773.

Fortina P, Kricka LJ, Surrey S, Grodzinski P. Nanobiotechnology: the promise and reality of new approaches to molecular recognition. Trends Biotechnol 2005;23:168-73.

Francois P, Bento M, Vaudaux P, Schrenzel J. Comparison of fluorescence and resonance light scattering for highly sensitive microarray detection of bacterial pathogens. J Microbiol Methods 2003;55:755-62.

Fritz J, Baller MK, Lang HP, et al. Translating biomolecular recognition into nanomechanics. Science 2000;288:316-8.

Gall JG, Pardue ML. Formation and detection of RNA-DNA hybrid molecules in cytological preparations. PNAS 1969;63:378-383.

Gao H, Shi W, Freund LB. Mechanics of receptor-mediated endocytosis. PNAS 2005;102:9469-74.

Georganopoulou DG, Chang L, Nam JM, et al. Nanoparticle-based detection in cerebral spinal fluid of a soluble pathogenic biomarker for Alzheimer's disease. PNAS 2005;102:2273-6.

Ghoroghchian PP, Frail PR, Susumu K, et al. Near-infrared-emissive polymersomes: Self-assembled soft matter for in vivo optical imaging. PNAS 2005;102:2922-7.

Gilbert B, Huang F, Zhang H, et al. Nanoparticles: Strained and Stiff. Science 2004;305:651-4.

Goodman CM, McCusker CD, Yilmaz T, Rotello VM. Toxicity of gold nanoparticles functionalized with cationic and anionic side chains. Bioconjug Chem 2004;15:897-900.

Gosalia DN, Diamond SL. Printing chemical libraries on microarrays for fluid phase nanoliter reactions. PNAS 2003;100:8721-6.

Grimm J, Manuel Perez J, Josephson L, Weissleder R. Novel Nanosensors for Rapid Analysis of Telomerase Activity. Cancer Research 2004;64:639-643.

Gupta A, Akin D, Bashir R. Single virus particle mass detection using microresonators with nanoscale thickness. Appl Phys Lett 2004;84: 1976-1978.

Gupta AK, Gupta M. Synthesis and surface engineering of iron oxide nanoparticles for biomedical applications. Biomaterials 2005 Jun;26:3995-4021.

Haase AT, Retzel EF, Staskus KA. Amplification and detection of lentiviral DNA inside cells. PNAS 1990;87:4971-4975.

Haes AJ, Duyne RP. Preliminary studies and potential applications of localized surface plasmon resonance spectroscopy in medical diagnostics. Expert Rev Mol Diagn 2004;4:527-37.

Hahm J, Lieber CM. Direct Ultrasensitive Electrical Detection of DNA and DNA Sequence Variations Using Nanowire Nanosensors. Nano Letters 2004;4:51-54.

Hamad-Schifferli K, Schwartz JJ, Santos AT, et al. Remote electronic control of DNA hybridization through inductive coupling to an attached metal nanocrystal antenna. Nature 2002;415:152-155.

Harisinghani MG, Barentsz J, Hahn PF, et al. Noninvasive detection of clinically occult lymph-node metastases in prostate cancer. N Engl J Med. 2003;348:2491-9.

Haruyama T. Micro- and nanobiotechnology for biosensing cellular responses. Adv Drug Deliv Rev 2003;55:393-401.

Hazarika P, Ceyhan B, Niemeyer CM. Reversible Switching of DNA-Gold Nanoparticle Aggregation. Angewandte Chemie International 2004;43:6469- 6471.

Higuchi R, Fockler C, Dollinger G, Watson R. Kinetic PCR analysis: real-time monitoring of DNA amplification reactions. Biotechnology (N Y) 1993;11:1026-30.

Hong BJ, Sunkara V, Park JW. DNA microarrays on nanoscale-controlled surface. Nucleic Acids Res 2005;33:e106

Howarth M, Takao K, Hayashi Y, Ting AY. Targeting quantum dots to surface proteins in living cells with biotin ligase. PNAS 2005 ;102:7583-8.

Howorka S, Cheley S, Bayley H. Sequence-specific detection of individual DNA strands using engineered nanopores. Nat Biotechnol 2001;19:636-9.

Hsu HY, Huang YY. RCA combined nanoparticle-based optical detection technique for protein microarray: a novel approach. Biosens Bioelectron 2004;20:123-6.

Ihara T, Tanaka S, Chikaura Y, Jyo A. Preparation of DNA-modified nanoparticles and preliminary study for colorimetric SNP analysis using their selective aggregations. Nucleic Acids Research 2004;32: e105.

Iijima S, Ajayan PM, Ichihashi T. Growth model for carbon nanotubes. Phys Rev Lett 1992;69:3100-3103.

Ishii D, Kinbara K, Ishida Y, et al. Chaperonin-mediated stabilization and ATP-triggered release of semiconductor nanoparticles. Nature 2003;423:628–632.

Jain KK. Applications of biochip and microarrays systems in pharmacogenomics. Pharmacogenomics 2000;1: 289-307.

Jain KK. Biochips for gene spotting. Science 2001;294:621-623.

Jain KK. Current Status of Fluorescent In Situ Hybridization. Medical Device Technology 2004;15:14-17.

Jain KK. Nanodiagnostics: application of nanotechnology in molecular diagnostics. Expert Rev Mol Diagn 2003a;4:153-161.

Jain KK. Current status of molecular biosensors. Medical Device Technology 2003b;14:10-5.

Jain KK. Current status of molecular biosensors. Medical Device Technology 2003;14:10-5.

Jain KK. Molecular Diagnostics: Technologies, Markets & Companies, Jain PharmaBiotech Publications, Basel, Switzerland, 2005.

Jain KK. Nanobiotechnology: Applications, Markets & Companies, Jain PharmaBiotech Publications, Basel, Switzerland, 2005b.

Jain KK. Nanotechnology in Clinical Laboratory Diagnostics. Clinica Chimica Acta 2005c;354:37-54.

Jain KK. Nanotechnology-based Lab-on-a-Chip Devices. In, Encyclopedia of Diagnostic Genomics and Proteomics, Marcel Dekkar Inc, New York, 2005d:891-895.

Jain KK. Proteomics: technologies, companies and markets. Jain PharmaBiotech Publications, Basel, Switzerland, 2005a.

Jain KK. The role of nanobiotechnology in drug discovery. Drug Discovery Today 2005e November 1;10: (in press).

Jaiswal JK, Goldman ER, Mattoussi H, Simon SM. Use of quantum dots for live cell imaging. Nature Methods 2004;1: 73 - 78.

Jaiswal JK, Mattoussi H, Mauro JM, Simon SM. Long-term multiple color imaging of live cells using quantum dot bioconjugates. Nat Biotechnol 2003;21:47-51.

Jia-Ming L, Hui ZG, Aihong W, et al. Determination of human IgG by solid substrate room temperature phosphorescence immunoassay based on an antibody labeled with nanoparticles containing Rhodamine 6G luminescent molecules. Spectrochim Acta A Mol Biomol Spectrosc 2005;61:923-7.

Karanikolos GP, Alexandridis P, Itskos G, et al. Synthesis and Size Control of Luminescent ZnSe Nanocrystals by a Microemulsion-Gas Contacting Technique. Langmuir 2004;20:550-553.

Karhanek M, Kemp JT, Pourmand N, et al. Single DNA Molecule Detection Using Nanopipettes and Nanoparticles. Nano Lett 2005;5:403 -407.

Kasianowicz JJ. Nanometer-scale pores: potential applications for analyte detection and DNA characterization. Dis Markers 2002;18:185-91.

Kim P, Lieber CM. Nanotube nanotweezers. Science 1999;286:2148-50.

Kircher MF, Mahmood U, King RS, et al. A Multimodal Nanoparticle for Preoperative Magnetic Resonance Imaging and Intraoperative Optical Brain Tumor Delineation. Cancer Research 2003;63:8122-8125.

Kobayashi H, Kawamoto S, Sakai Y, et al. Lymphatic drainage imaging of breast cancer in mice by micro-magnetic resonance lymphangiography using a nano-size paramagnetic contrast agent. J Natl Cancer Inst 2004;96:703-8.

Köhler G and Milstein C. Continuous cultures of fused cells secreting antibody of predefined specificity. Nature 1975;256:495-497.

Komiyama S, Astafiev O, Antonov H, et al. A single-photon detector in the far-infrared range. Nature 2000;403:405-7.

Koskinen JO, Vaarno J, Meltola NJ, et al. Fluorescent nanoparticles as labels for immunometric assay of C-reactive protein using two-photon excitation assay technology. Anal Biochem 2004;328:210-8.

Kumar R, Singh SK, Koshkin AA, et al. The first analogues of LNA (locked nucleic acids): phosphorothioate-LNA and 2'-thio-LNA. Bioorg Med Chem Lett 1998;8:2219-22.

Lang MJ, Fordyce PM, Block SM. Combined optical trapping and single-molecule fluorescence. Journal of Biology 2003;2(1):6 (http://jbiol.com/content/2/1/6).

Larson DR, Zipfel WR, Williams RM, et al. Water-Soluble Quantum Dots for Multiphoton Fluorescence Imaging in Vivo. Science 2003;300:1434-1436.

Legleiter J, Czilli DL, Gitter B, et al. Effect of different anti-Abeta antibodies on Abeta fibrillogenesis as assessed by atomic force microscopy. J Mol Biol 2004;335:997-1006.

Lehn JM. Supramolecular chemistry – scope and perspectives: molecules, supermolecules, and molecular devices. Ang Chem Int Ed Engl 1988;27:89-112.

Lichter P, Bayle AL, Cremer T& Ward DC. Analysis of genes and chromosomes by non-isotopic in situ hybridization. Genetic Analysis and Technical Applications 1991;8:24-35.

Llinás RR, Walton KD, Nakao M, et al. Neuro-vascular central nervous recording/stimulating system: Using nanotechnology probes. Journal of Nanoparticle Research 2005;7:111-127.

Lyuksyutov IF, Naugle DG, Rathnayaka KDD. On-chip manipulation of levitated femtodroplets. Applied Physics Letters 2004;85:1817-1819.

Matsunaga T, Okamura Y. Genes and proteins involved in bacterial magnetic particle formation. Trends Microbiol. 2003;11:536-41.

McKendry R, Zhang J, Arntz Y, et al. Multiple label-free biodetection and quantitative DNA-binding assays on a nanomechanical cantilever array. PNAS 2002;99:9783-8.

McKenzie JL, Waid MC, Shi R, Webster TJ. Decreased functions of astrocytes on carbon nanofiber materials. Biomaterials. 2004;25:1309-17.

McShane MJ. Potential for glucose monitoring with nanoengineered fluorescent biosensors. Diabetes Technol Ther 2002;4:533-8.

Medintz IL, Uyeda HT, Goldman ER, Mattoussi H. Quantum dot bioconjugates for imaging, labelling and sensing. Nat Mater 2005 Jun;4:435-46.

Melechko AV, McKnight TE, Guillorn MA, et al. Nanopipe fabrication using vertically aligned carbon nanofiber templates. Journal of Vacuum Science & Technology B: Microelectronics and Nanometer Structures 2002;20:2730-2733.

Meng G, Jung YJ, Cao A, et al. Controlled fabrication of hierarchically branched nanopores, nanotubes, and nanowires. PNAS 2005;102:7074-8.

Merrifield CJ, Perrais D, Zenisek D. Coupling between Clathrin-Coated-Pit Invagination, Cortactin Recruitment, and Membrane Scission Observed in Live Cells. Cell 2005:121:593-606.

Michalet X, Pinaud FF, Bentolila LA, et al. Quantum dots for live cells, in vivo imaging, and diagnostics. Science 2005;307:538-44.

Mullis K, Faloona F, Scharf S, et al. Specific enzymatic amplification of DNA in vitro: the polymerase chain reaction. Cold Spring Harbor Symposium on Quantitative Biology 1986;51:263-273.

Munge B, Liu G, Collins G, Wang J. Multiple enzyme layers on carbon nanotubes for electrochemical detection down to 80 DNA copies. Anal Chem 2005 Jul 15;77:4662-6.

Myhra S. A review of enabling technologies based on scanning probe microscopy relevant to bioanalysis. Biosens Bioelectron. 2004;19:1345-54.

Nam JM, Stoeva SI, Mirkin CA. Bio-Bar-Code-Based DNA Detection with PCR-like Sensitivity. J Am Chem Soc 2004;126:5932-5933.

Nam JM, Thaxton CS, Mirkin CA. Nanoparticle-Based Bio-Bar Codes for the Ultrasensitive Detection of Proteins. Science 2003;301:1884-1886.

Neuwelt EA, Varallyay P, Bago AG, et al. Imaging of iron oxide nanoparticles by MR and light microscopy in patients with malignant brain tumours. Neuropathology and Applied Neurobiology 2004;30:456-71.

Nicewarner-Pena SR, Freeman RG, Reiss BD, et al. Submicrometer metallic barcodes. Science 2001;294:137-41.

Niemeyer CM. Semi-synthetic DNA-protein conjugates: novel tools in analytics and nanobiotechnology. Biochem Soc Trans 2004;32(Pt 1):51-3.

Oberle V, Bakowsky U, Hoekstra D. Lipoplex assembly visualized by atomic force microscopy. Methods Enzymol. 2003;373:281-97.

Oberringer M, Englisch A, Heinz B, et al. Atomic force microscopy and scanning near-field optical microscopy studies on the characterization of human metaphase chromosomes. Eur Biophys J 2003;32:620-7.

Okumoto S, Looger LL, Micheva KD, et al. Detection of glutamate release from neurons by genetically encoded surface-displayed FRET nanosensors. PNAS 2005;102:8740-5.

Ozkan M. Quantum dots and other nanoparticles: what can they offer to drug discovery? Drug Discov Today 2004;9:1065-71.

Park SJ, Taton TA, Mirkin CA. Array-based electrical detection of DNA with nanoparticle probes. Science 2002;295:1503-6.

Patolsky F, Zheng G, Hayden O, et al. Electrical detection of single viruses. PNAS 2004;101:14017-14022.

Pei J, Tian F, Thundat T. Glucose biosensor based on the microcantilever. Anal Chem. 2004;76:292-7.

Perez JM, Simeone FJ, Saeki Y, Josephson L, Weissleder R. Viral-induced self-assembly of magnetic nanoparticles allows the detection of viral particles in biological media. J Am Chem Soc 2003;12510192-3.

Piner RD, Zhu J, Xu F, Hong S, Mirkin CA. Dip-pen nanolithography. Science 1999;283:661- 663.

Pinkel D, Gray JW, Trask B, et al. Cytogenetic analysis by in situ hybridization with fluorescently labeled nucleic acid probes. Cold Spring Harb Symp Quant Biol 1986;51 Pt 1:151-7.

Qu X, Wu D, Mets L, Scherer NF. Nanometer-localized multiple single-molecule fluorescence microscopy. PNAS 2004;101:11298-303.

Reichert J, Csaki A, Kohler JM, Fritzsche W. Chip-based optical detection of DNA hybridization by means of nanobead labeling. Anal Chem 2000;72:6025-9.

Reimer P, Bremer C, Allkemper T, et al. Myocardial perfusion and MR angiography of chest with SH U 555 C: results of placebo-controlled clinical phase I study. Radiology. 2004;231:474-81.

Riehn R, Lu M, Wang YM, et al. Restriction mapping in nanofluidic devices. PNAS 2005 Jul 19;102:10012-6.

Roco MC. Nanotechnology: convergence with modern biology and medicine. Curr Opin Biotechnol. 2003;14:337-46.

Rosario R, Gust JD, Garcia AA, et al. Lotus Effect Amplifies Light-Induced Contact Angle Switching. J Phys Chem B 2004; 108; 12640-12642.

Salata O. Applications of nanoparticles in biology and medicine. Journal of Nanobiotechnology 2004;2:3.

Saleh A, Schroeter M, Jonkmanns C, et al. In vivo MRI of brain inflammation in human ischaemic stroke. Brain 2004;127(Pt 7):1670-7.

Santangelo PJ, Nix B, Tsourkas A, Bao G. Dual FRET molecular beacons for mRNA detection in living cells. Nucleic Acids Research 2004;32(6): e57.

Saunders NA, Alexander S, Tatt I. env Gene typing of human immunodeficiency virus type 1 strains on electronic microarrays. J Clin Microbiol 2005;43:1910-6.

Schmidt J, Montemagno C: Using machines in cells. Drug Discov Today 2002;7:500-503.

Schmieder AH, Winter PM, Caruthers SD, et al. Molecular MR imaging of melanoma angiogenesis with anb3-targeted paramagnetic nanoparticles. Magnetic Resonance in Medicine 2005;53:621-627.

Seydack M. Nanoparticle labels in immunosensing using optical detection methods. Biosens Bioelectron 2005 Jun 15;20:2454-69.

Shapiro EM, Skrtic S, Sharer K, et al. MRI detection of single particles for cellular imaging. PNAS 2004;101:10901-6.

Singh-Zocchi M, Dixit S, Ivanov V, Zocchi G. Single-molecule detection of DNA hybridization. PNAS 2003;100:7605-10.

Sinton D. Microscale flow visualization. Microfluidics and Nanofluidics 2004;1:2-21.

Sirbuly DJ, Law M, Pauzauskie P, et al. Optical routing and sensing with nanowire assemblies. PNAS 2005;102:7800-7805.

Sleytr UB, Sara M, Messner P, Pum D. Two-dimensional protein crystals (S-layers): fundamentals and applications. J Cell Biochem 1994;56:171-6.

Smalley RE. In, Bartlett RJ (ed) Comparison of Ab Initio Quantum Chemistry with Experiments for Small Molecules. D. Riedel, Boston, 1985.

Smith CH, Tondra M. Magnetoresistive Detection of Flowing and Immobilized Assay Labels. Nanomaterials 2004 Nanobiotechnology and Nanomedicine Conference, 27 October 2004, Stamford, Conn, USA.

Srinivas PR, Barker P, Srivastava S. Nanotechnology in early detection of cancer. Lab Invest 2002;82:657-62.

Storhoff JJ, Lucas AD, Garimella V, Bao YP, Müller UR. Homogeneous detection of unamplified genomic DNA sequences based on colorimetric scatter of gold nanoparticle probes. Nat Biotech 2004;22: 883-7.

Stroh C, Wang H, Bash R, et al. Single-molecule recognition imaging microscopy. PNAS 2004;101:12503-7.

Sukhanova A, Devy J, Venteo L, et al. Biocompatible fluorescent nanocrystals for immunolabeling of membrane proteins and cells. Anal Biochem 2004;324:60-7.

Sumner JP, Aylott JW, Monson E, Kopelman R. A fluorescent PEBBLE nanosensor for intracellular free zinc. Analyst 2002;127:11-6.

Tabuchi M, Ueda M, Kaji N, Yamasaki Y, et al. Nanospheres for DNA separation chips. Nat Biotechnol 2004;22:337-340.

Tan M, Wang G, Hai X, et al. Development of functionalized fluorescent europium nanoparticles for biolabeling and time-resolved fluorometric applications. Journal of Materials Chemistry 2004;14:2896-2901.

Tomalia DA, Baker H, Dewald J, et al. A new class of polymers: starburst-dendritic macromolecules. Polym J 1985;17:117-132.

Urdea MS, Wilber JC, Yeghiazarian T, et al. Direct and quantitative detection of HIV-1 RNA in human plasma with a branched DNA signal amplification assay. AIDS 1993;7 Suppl 2:S11-4.

Valanne A, Huopalahti S, Soukka T, et al. A sensitive adenovirus immunoassay as a model for using nanoparticle label technology in virus diagnostics. J Clin Virol 2005 Jul;33:217-23.

van de Goor T. Nanopore detection: threading DNA through a tiny hole. PharmacoGenomics 2004 March/April: pp. 28-29.

Venne K, Bonneil E, Eng K, Thibault P. Enhanced Sensitivity in Proteomics Analyses Using NanoLC–MS and high-field asymmetry waveform ion mobility mass spectrometry. Anal Chem 2005;77:2176-86.

Voura EB, Jaiswal JK, Mattoussi H, Simon SM. Tracking metastatic tumor cell extravasation with quantum dot nanocrystals and fluorescence emission-scanning microscopy. Nat Med 2004;10:993-8.

Walton ID, Norton SM, Balasingham A, et al. Particles for multiplexed analysis in solution: detection and identification of striped metallic particles using optical microscopy. Anal Chem 2002;74:2240-7.

Wang WU, Chen C, Lin K, et al. Label-free detection of small-molecule-protein interactions by using nanowire nanosensors. PNAS 2005;102:3208–3212.

Watson JD, Crick FHC. Genetic implications of the structure of deoxyribonucleic acid. Nature 1953;171:964-969.

Weeks BL, Camarero J, Noy A, et al. A microcantilever-based pathogen detector. Scanning 2003;25:297-9.

Weston AD, Hood L. Systems biology, proteomics, and the future of health care: toward predictive, preventative, and personalized medicine. J Proteome Res 2004;3:179-96.

Won J, Kim M, Yi YW, et al. A magnetic nanoprobe technology for detecting molecular interactions in live cells. Science. 2005 Jul 1;309:121-5.

Wu G, Datar RH, Hansen KM, et al. Bioassay of prostate-specific antigen (PSA) using microcantilevers. Nature Biotechnology 2001;19:856–860.

Wu X, Liu H, Liu J, et al. Immunofluorescent labeling of cancer marker Her2 and other cellular targets with semiconductor quantum dots. Nat Biotechnol 2003;21:41-6.

Yan H, He R, Johnson J, et al. Dendritic nanowire ultraviolet laser array. J Am Chem Soc 2003;125:4728-9.

Yang L, Li Y. Quantum dots as fluorescent labels for quantitative detection of Salmonella typhimurium in chicken carcass wash water. J Food Prot 2005 Jun;68:1241-5.

Yang W, Zhang CG, Qu HY, et al. Novel fluorescent silica nanoparticle probe for ultrasensitive immunoassays. Anal Chim Acta 2004;503:163–169.

Yguerabide J, Yguerabide EE. Resonance light scattering particles as ultrasensitive labels for detection of analytes in a wide range of applications. J Cell Biochem Suppl 2001;Suppl 37:71-81.

Zhao X, Hilliard LR, Mechery SJ, et al. A rapid bioassay for single bacterial cell quantitation using bioconjugated nanoparticles. PNAS 2004;101:15027-32.

Zuiderwijk M, Tanke HJ, Sam Niedbala R, Corstjens PL. An amplification-free hybridization-based DNA assay to detect Streptococcus pneumoniae utilizing the up-converting phosphor technology. Clin Biochem 2003;36:401-3.

INDEX

Books of Related Interest

Full details of all these books at: www.horizonpress.com